Maternal–Child Home Health Aide Training Manual

Maternal–Child Home Health Aide Training Manual

Mary Ann Chestnut, RN

President, Citadel MCH, Inc.
Narberth, Pennsylvania

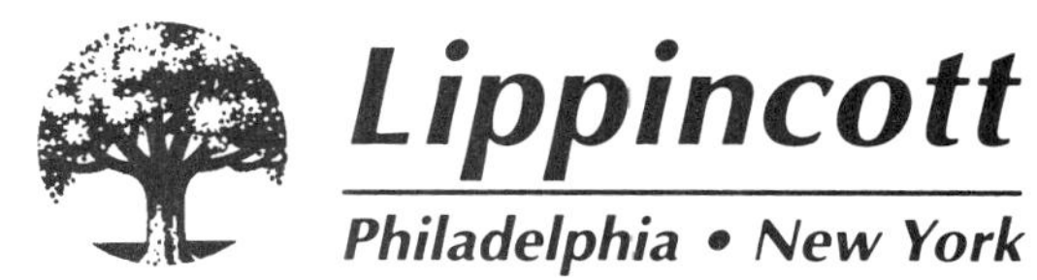

Acquisitions Editor: Jennifer E. Brogan
Coordinating Editorial Assistant: Susan V. Barta
Production Editor: Virginia Barishek
Production Manager: Helen Ewan
Production Service: Berliner Inc.
Printer/Binder: Victor Graphics
Cover Designer: Joan Wendt
Cover Printer: Lehigh Press

9 8 7 6 5 4 3 2 1

Library of Congress Cataloging-in-Publication Data

Chestnut, Mary Ann
Maternal–child home health aide training manual / Mary Ann Chestnut.
p. cm.
Includes bibliographical references and index.
ISBN 0-7817-1204-1
1. Home health aides—Training of—Handbooks, manuals, etc. 2. Maternal health services—Handbooks, manuals, etc. 3. Child health services—Handbooks, manuals, etc. I. Title.
[DNLM: 1. Home Health Aides. 2. Maternal Health Services. 3. Child Health Services. W 21.5 C525m 1997]
RA645.3.C475 1997
362.1'982—dc21
DNLM/DLC
for Library of Congress 97-25845
CIP

Care has been taken to confirm the accuracy of the information presented and to describe generally accepted practices. However, the authors, editors, and publisher are not responsible for errors or omissions or for any consequences from application of the information in this book and make no warranty, express or implied, with respect to the contents of the publication.

The authors, editors and publisher have exerted every effort to ensure that drug selection and dosage set forth in this text are in accordance with current recommendations and practice at the time of publication. However, in view of ongoing research, changes in government regulations, and the constant flow of information relating to drug therapy and drug reactions, the reader is urged to check the package insert for each drug for any change in indications and dosages and for added warnings and precautions. This is particularly important when the recommended agent is a new or infrequently employed drug.

Some drugs and medical devices presented in this publication have Food and Drug Administration (FDA) clearance for limited use in restricted research settings. It is the responsibility of the health care provider to ascertain the FDA status of each drug or device planned for use in their clinical practice.

This book is dedicated to Ellen Craighead, RN, BSN, Lucille Perna, RN, BSN, and Roberta Capewell, RN, MSN, who together gave me the challenge to develop and implement a home health aide program targeted to serve maternal–child families; and to the mothers on the 1992–1995 Pennsylvania statewide task force on maternal–child home and community-based services, all of whom were former clients who volunteered their time to help develop the standards by speaking out on the need:

Eileen Bellinger
Barbara Bellinger
Theresa Lewis
Carmen Sharp
Josephine Nyame
Kyme McCleary

And finally to Sister Theresita Hinnegan, RN, CNM, whose commitment to maternal–child health care in the community has been an inspiration to so very many.

One percent of the author's royalties from the sale of this book will be donated by the author to the startup of a nonprofit nursing center to advance the practice of maternal–child home health.

Preface

The purpose of this book is to provide a resource for the vast array of providers currently offering or desiring to integrate paraprofessional service programs for the maternal–child population. The importance of the paraprofessional in providing care to the client at home is often overlooked, especially in maternal–child health. The job titles of paraprofessionals vary with the organization providing the care. In Medicare-certified agencies, this role is usually titled "home health aide" or "personal care assistant." Hospital-based programs and community-based facilities may refer to this person as a "lay home visitor." Regardless of the classification, paraprofessional support in the home has provided effective service in many organizational settings. Many insurance companies have active perinatal management programs that use home health aides as an alternative to hospitalization for women with high-risk pregnancies who must remain on bedrest and who lack adequate help at home.

The use of home health aides for disabled children has grown tremendously as federal laws have evolved over the past 10 years to prevent out-of-home placement despite the family's inability to provide care 24 hours a day. For children with developmental delays or disabilities (physical or mental), federal law also provides entitlement for early intervention services that may be provided in the home or within a center, depending on the child's age and condition. Services for which funding is available through this entitlement include both home care for the child and respite care for the primary caregivers. Paraprofessional services are often a part of this service plan.

The demand for paraprofessional caregivers has also grown significantly in programs that strive to reduce infant mortality. These services are typically referred to as "lay home visiting." Lay home visitors provide home visits for at-risk pregnant women or at-risk infants. Federally funded studies have found that lay home visitors are effective in reducing infant mortality within high-risk groups such as pregnant adolescents and infants born with drug exposure. Lay home visitors are used in both rural and urban settings.

All of these services and paraprofessional titles have one primary thing in common: They all require well-trained, qualified individuals. As a result of the rapid expansion of paraprofessional services, providers often lack a resource for training persons to work in maternal–child health. This book seeks to fill the gap. *Maternal–Child Home Health Aide Training Manual* will be a vital tool to any organization providing in-home services to pregnant women, infants, and children.

The manual offers the basic components necessary to any maternal–child home health aide training program. Chapter 1 presents the personnel policies for any program, including pertinent job descriptions. Chapter 2 contains standards to be used in the training program. These standards have been developed to address Medicare conditions of participation for home health agencies and standards of the Joint Commission on the Accreditation of Health Organizations; however, all types of providers will find them helpful. Chapter 3 offers a series of modules to be used as teaching tools in the training program. The modules were developed to provide a basic training standard requirement for all paraprofessionals providing maternal–child services. The learning modules include safety (child and household), household management, infection control, communication, care of the pregnant and postpartum woman, and care of the newborn. Organizations can use these modules as a core curriculum for all paraprofessionals and expand upon them to address more complex areas of care. Chapter 4 contains educational and informational handouts that can be copied and given to staff and client as teaching tools. The appendix contains personnel records, competency tests, clinical records, and basic policies and procedures for taking vital signs that can be used in the training program. The Appendix is followed by a list of abbreviations and a glossary. A bibliography that providers will find useful for educational resources is also included. With the growing emphasis on cost containment in health care, we can only expect to see a greater need for paraprofessional services. Providers must be ready to respond.

This book evolved through years of research, development, and actual implementation of maternal–child paraprofessional programs provided both in urban and rural counties of Pennsylvania by Citadel MCH Services and Family Help, Inc. Citadel MCH Services at this writing had been licensed and Medicare certified as a home health agency by the Pennsylvania Department of Health for 4 years.

Family Help, Inc. was similarly licensed and certified as a home health agency in addition to having been awarded accreditation by the Joint Commission on the Accreditation of Health Care organizations. Both companies exclusively provided maternal–child health care.

Mary Ann Chestnut, RN

Acknowledgments

As a nurse working in the field of maternal-child health since 1982, I have had the privilege of working with many individuals who contributed to my knowledge and inspired me to write and publish this manuscript. I would like to thank and acknowledge those who have so willingly contributed this support.

- *The staff of Booth Maternity Center, Philadelphia, Pennsylvania, who are too numerous to list here.*

- *The staff at Family Help, Inc., including:*
  Ellen Craighead, RN, BSN
  Marilyn Kerr, RN, BSN
  Bonnie Charleston
  Anne Ravdin, RN, BSN
  Ann Galanter, RN, BSN
  Joanne Fischer, MSW
  Laurie Reardon, RN, BSN
  Barbara Tinus, RN, BSN
  Gail Pierson, RN, PNP
  Barbara Krinsky, RN, BSN
  Millie Boettcher, RN, MSN
  Patricia Larsen, RN, MSN, CNM
  Debbie Westcott, RN, BSN
  Judy Woomer, CHHA
  and all the other staff who made Family Help a reality

- *The staff at Citadel MCH Services*
  Sonya Newell Wilson, RN
  Kathleen Whalen, RN
  Jacqueline Williams, RN, BSN
  Vicki Newell
  Carol Hallenback, RN, BSN
  Judy Podosky, RNC
  Ann Galanter, RN, BS
  Norma Cintron, RN

- *Also a joint acknowledgment must be made to those who served on The Professional Advisory Committees of Family Help, Inc. (1985–1990) and/or The Professional Advisory Committees of Citadel MCH Services, Inc. (1991–1995):*
  Paul Branca, MD
  Ronald Bolognese, MD
  Judy Bernbaum, MD
  Evelyn Bouden, MD
  Carl Bailey
  Jannie L. Blackwell
  Roberta Capewell, RN, MSN, PNP
  Julia Clarke, RN, CNM, MSN
  Jane Eleey, MSW
  Jeffrey Gerdes, MD
  Page Talbott Gould, PhD
  Howard Grant, MD, JD
  Robert Holmes, MD
  Susan Hutchinson, RNC, MSN
  Mark A. Kalchbrenner, DO
  Rich Kaplan, MD
  June Kinney, PhD
  Rose Kinney, RN, BSN
  Judith McCoyd, ACSW, LSW
  Carol L. Natter, PT
  Lucille Pema, RN, BSN
  Albert Pizzica, DO
  Barbara Ritchey, ACSW, LSW
  Jeffrey Rothirtan, EdD:, PT
  Barbara Schraeder, RN, PhD
  Robert Stavis, PhD, MD
  Patricia Thiebault, RD
  Barbara Wesley, MD, MPH
  Robert S. Wimmer, MD
  Mary Wright, MOT
  Susan Yates, CNM, MSN

- *I also want to thank Scott Bucher, RN and Mylo Woodward, RN of the Pennsylvania Department of Health, Maternal–Child Division, and Frank Heron of the U.S. Department of Health and Human Services for their support and assistance throughout the years.*

Contents

CHAPTER 3

Home Health Aide Training Modules 25

CHAPTER 4

Home Health Aide–Family Teaching Materials 87

CHAPTER 1

Personnel Policies and Procedures

This chapter covers the basic personnel policies and procedures necessary for a quality health care service program. The job descriptions detail qualifications, duties, and responsibilities of the Home Health Aide. In addition, requirements for professional nurse supervision are also included. Clearly, one of the first responsibilities of any training instructor is to assure that the trainee has a good understanding of the job. The contents of this chapter will be helpful through the recruitment and orientation process to define roles and measure expected performance requirements. The nurse and the Home Health Aide are a team in the provision of care and as such should understand how their roles combine to offer the family an effective plan that meets their individual needs.

RECRUITMENT, TRAINING, AND SUPERVISION OF HOME HEALTH AIDES

POLICY:

Home health aides are selected with many factors in mind, such as a sympathetic attitude toward care of the sick, the ability to read, write, and carry out directions, maturity, and the ability to deal effectively with the demands of the job. They are closely supervised to ensure their competence in providing care. The home health agency must use individuals who meet the personnel qualifications specified in the Medicare conditions for Home Health Aides. In addition, agencies should verify additional requirements of the individual state with their state home health association, their state home health licensing agency, or their state Medicare office. Additional requirements may include criminal background checks or child abuse clearance. The agency will designate responsibility to the supervising nurse and program instructor to remain current on changes in Medicare, state, and local requirements for personnel and to integrate these changes as needed to written policy and procedure.

PURPOSE:

Selection, training, and supervision policies and procedures are designed to assure provision of safe and appropriate care to patients by appropriately qualified Home Health Aides.

PROCEDURE:

Each Home Health Aide is an employee of the agency (part-time if working less than 40 hours a week), and all employee policies as outlined for Home Health Aides and staff in general will apply.

An employment agreement and a current personnel file must be completed before the probation period can be satisfactorily completed. The probation period begins at the time of the first case accepted by the aide and continues until 300 hours of work are completed. It is expected that all aides will comply with all agency goals, philosophies, and policies in carrying out their duties.

Home health aides are neat, clean, and professional in appearance; report to work promptly and without fail; notify the agency in a timely manner when a delay or absence is expected; complete the appropriate paperwork for the agency and for patient care needs; remain flexible in scheduling and changing of cases; act professionally and considerately in the homes of patients; and provide the highest quality of services to clients.

The training program consists of 80 hours of instruction. All aides must be CPR-certified. Chapter 2 outlines the training program. Successful completion of this course includes attendance at classes, completion of all assigned work, satisfactory demonstration of procedures, satisfactory completion of written, verbal, and practical examinations, and a satisfactory review by the training instructor.

SPECIFIC DUTIES OF THE HOME HEALTH AIDE

The Home Health Aide is responsible for participating in the development and implementation of the care plan. This includes the following responsibilities.

1. Complete environmental assessment. Identify safety and health hazards to charge nurse and other team members. Correct safety and health deficiencies or supervise their correction. Communicate any safety hazards for aide to agency.

2. Complete family assessment.

3. Maintain a safe, healthy, and clean household, including cleaning living/dining area, kitchen, bathroom, and bedrooms according to plan.
   a. Cleaning includes running vacuum, dusting, dry or wet mopping, and straightening and picking up area.
   b. Cleaning also includes scrubbing/waxing floors, washing windows, shampooing carpets, and cleaning cupboards and/or closets on a routine schedule.
   c. Doing laundry and ironing clothing as needed, as well as changing and laundering bed linens daily, are also important responsibilities.

4. Support social and emotional needs of child/family.
   a. Attempt to keep household running as normally as possible.
   b. Practice effective listening and communication techniques.
   c. Maintain patient and family as center of planning and work.
   d. Identify abnormal/aberrant behavior and report to supervisor.
   e. Shop for food, and prepare and serve nutritious meals.
      1) Aide is required to purchase food as directed by the family if they provide transportation and money.
      2) Aide is required to plan, prepare, serve, and clean up after meals that are part of the plan of care. Aide should also prepare nutritious snacks as appropriate.

5. Teach and serve as role model as needed.
   a. Aide is required to teach any family members the appropriate care of self, cleaning house/laundry, preparation of food, and procedures that are involved in child care and that family members will have to assume once the aide is no longer present or during other times of care.
   b. Aide should consistently teach the child and family good and safe health practices.

6. Provide patient care.
   a. Take vital signs and blood pressure, report abnormals, and record all information.
   b. Keep track of food intake and appetite, recording same; maintain accurate intake and output when ordered and document this information.
   c. Perform personal care as appropriate, such as bathing, hair care, oral hygiene, routine skin care, turning, and positioning.
   d. Perform range of motion exercises according to care plan.

e. Assist patient with lifting, moving, turning, and ambulating; measure patient as directed.
f. Make bed and change linens.
g. Assist with excretory function as appropriate.
h. Assist with changing clothes.
i. Monitor fluid and salt intake as well as follow special diet instructions.
j. Attend to indwelling catheter.
k. Collect specimens for routine and C&S urine, 24-hour urine, stool collection, straining urine.
l. Administer enemas as directed.
m. Care for perineal area PRN.
n. Assist with deep breathing and coughing exercises.
o. Change dressing (sterile, packing, soaks).
p. Assist with application of bandages and dressings.
q. Manage urine and blood testing for diabetics.
r. Assist mother with uterine monitor transmissions.
s. Provide support for the patient and family during illness.
t. Observe patient condition, noting changes and abnormals and reporting and recording all information.
u. Report and record any untoward events, attitudes, symptoms, etc.
v. Provide first aid in cases of accidental injury.
w. Provide simple aid for cuts and bruises.
x. Maintain regular communication with charge nurse regarding any problems, questions, or untoward events.
y. Observe for any aberrant social situations and report them.
z. Maintain good infection control techniques in every area of work.

7. Provide infant/child care, which includes the following responsibilities.
   a. Bathe infant/child.
   b. Perform routine mouth care.
   c. Measure infant as indicated.
   d. Feed infant/child.
   e. Monitor intake and output as well as appetite.
   f. Supervise infant/child throughout the day.
   g. Provide safe, healthful environment for play and sleep.
   h. Maintain normal schedule as much as possible.
   i. Stimulate infant/child development through exercises and activities.
   j. Encourage physical development appropriate to age level.

8. Manage certain technical care.
   a. Supervise and observe intravenous therapy, noting and reporting problems.
   b. Manage care of the infant on the apnea monitor according to protocol.
   c. Manage care of the sick child according to care plan.
   d. Manage ostomy care.
   e. Manage gastrostomy feeding.
   f. Manage restraints when needed.
   g. Manage cast care.
   h. Manage care of the patient in traction.
   i. Manage care of the infant/child in a croupette or oxygen tank.
   j. Manage care of the infant/child receiving oxygen.
   k. Manage care of infant/child requiring periodic suctioning.
   l. Provide maintenance care: ordering and supervising the use of needed supplies and equipment.
9. Maintain effective infection control.
   a. Assure personal cleanliness.
   b. Practice proper handwashing techniques.
   c. Maintain clean/sterile procedures as appropriate.
   d. Teach family about infection control.
10. Handle any emergencies that arise.
    a. Know how to identify an emergency.
    b. Provide appropriate emergency care.
    c. The Home Health Aide must be CPR-certified and first-aid-certified.
11. Clear, concise, timely reporting and recording of all information.
    a. Maintain communication with supervisor.
    b. Report all untoward events.
    c. Record all care and work performed.
    d. Maintain agency records.

ASSIGNMENT AND SUPERVISION OF THE HOME HEALTH AIDE

POLICY: Home health aides will receive assignments from a registered nurse in a clearly written format.

PROCEDURE: The registered nurse will prepare written instructions for patient care on a Home Health Aide Care Plan, which is contained as part of the medical record of the agency.

The registered nurse will make a supervisory visit to the patient's residence at least every 2 weeks. The registered nurse will call the patient before each visit, which will occur either when the aide is present to observe and assist or when the aide is absent. It is recommended that the initial visit take place when the aide is present to assure appropriate understanding of the initial instructions for patient care. It is then recommended that the registered nurse providing supervision of patient care shall contact the patient within the first week of service to assess overall satisfaction with care and schedule a supervisory visit that will occur when the Home Health Aide is absent to assess relationships and determine whether the goals of care are being met.

Following the supervisory visit, the registered nurse providing supervision will determine changes necessary based upon the evaluation, taking opportunities to improve both patient/family relationships and direct patient care. The registered nurse must make supervisory visits to the patient's residence at least every 2 weeks through the patient's entire term of care, for as long as Home Health Aide services are received from the agency.

The registered nurse shall document the supervisory visits on the clinical nursing progress note and record changes on the Home Health Aide Care Plan, reporting changes made as a result of the supervisory visit.

HOME HEALTH AIDE PROGRAM

Philosophy

The Home Health Agency believes that many home health care needs can be managed through the services of trained Home Health Aides with proper nursing supervision.

Goals of the Program

The goal of the Home Health Aide Program is to maintain a staff of well-trained and experienced Home Health Aides who are sensitive and intelligent and of high character to serve families in times of crisis and disruption due to health problems, to assist in the care of certain patients who can benefit from care at home as an alternative to hospitalization, to provide basic nursing care to patients whose care does not require professional nursing, and to provide cost-effective custodial care for total care patients.

Professional nursing staff members work collaboratively with the Home Health Aide in an effort to address all facets of the problems generated by a family member's illness.

Goals of Home Care

Goals for the home care of every patient are individualized. There are similar overall goals, however, for the care of all patients. The goals of the Home Health Aide Program are as follows.

1. Promote self-care and independence.
2. Assure safety and comfort.
3. Maintain dignity.
4. Maintain stability.

ROLE OF THE HOME HEALTH AIDE

The role of the Home Health Aide is to serve as a member of a team that consists of the physician, the agency nurse, the hospital discharge planner or social worker, the specialists, the agency scheduling staff, the community resource people, and the family members, and support people.

This team uses various methods to assess, develop, and organize a plan of home care based on diagnoses and physical needs as well as family and psychosocial needs, culture, and preferences. Additionally, the team provides technical and physical care, renders emotional and (at times) spiritual support, stabilizes the family situation through appropriate household management, and facilitates the use of community and other resources.

The Home Health Aide should be a mature, healthy, responsible, and conscientious man or woman who is compassionate, considerate, and experienced in life and health matters. He or she cares about and likes people, has a sensitivity to children and infants, and possesses special characteristics of patience, commitment, and sensitivity to the needs of those in emotional and physical pain. Home health aides must be particularly aware of family dynamics and have an understanding of the importance of the family in society and, therefore, have a concern for the maintenance of family life through crises and through the disruption created by illness of a family member.

HOME HEALTH AIDE JOB DESCRIPTION

Principal Functions

1. Provide assistance to the patient so he or she may achieve maximum self-reliance.
2. Prepare and serve of nutritious meals.
3. Provide support during particular events in the patient's life cycle, provide personal care according to the nursing care plan, and meet emotional needs.
4. Maintain a clean and healthful environment.
5. Report changes in the patient's condition.

Supervision

The Home Health Aide is supervised by a visiting registered nurse.

Qualifications

1. The aide must be of high moral character and have compassion for the sick and sensitivity to the family of the sick child or parent.
2. The aide must be caring and sensitive, willing to serve in the appropriate forum of care for each patient/family.
3. The aide must complete a Home Health Aide training course, documenting satisfactory completion of a minimum of 75 hours of training, or have passed the verbal, written, and practical examinations. All Home Health Aides must complete 16 or more hours of classroom training before performing patient care. Aides must take an additional 16 hours of practical training supervised by a qualified registered nurse.

Responsibilities

1. Receive supervision and assignment from the charge nurse.
2. Assist in development of and implementation of the care plan.
3. Establish the client/family relationship through development of a mutually agreed upon household management and care plan.
4. Explain all procedures and rationales to the client prior to performance.
5. Perform procedures listed as Home Health Aide duties according to an approved written nursing care plan or orders.
6. Report changes and untoward events to the charge nurse.
7. Assist the children and family members in making the transition to home life. Perform household organization activities and provide comfort and safety measures.
8. ***Do not*** administer medications.
9. Teach child/family and provide educational material as directed by the nursing supervisor.
10. Provide child care such as feeding, bathing, etc. as outlined in the care plan.
11. Prepare and assist with nutritious meals, incorporating special diets as prescribed.
12. Perform routine household tasks.
13. Maintain written documentation as required by the agency.
14. Complete required paperwork for scheduling, payroll, personnel files, etc.
15. Maintain confidentiality concerning all patient care and record keeping.
16. Document all care given, work completed, and observations, both subjective and objective; document all reports given and instructions received.
17. Attend required agency in-service training programs.

CHAPTER 2

Content of Training Program

This chapter deals with the actual policies and procedures of a training program for Home Health Aides or other paraprofessionals seeking to serve the health care needs of the maternal–child population. Included are job descriptions for instructors and competency evaluators, annual in-service requirements, minimum course competency requirements, and a suggested outline of subjects to be covered in training.

The minimum course competency requirements are those that must be taught in a federally certified agency. To achieve Medicare certification to provide Home Health Aide services, which is a frequent requirement for agencies to receive reimbursement from Medicaid and other third party insurers, training programs must include the minimum course competencies outlined in this chapter. Users may wish to modify the suggested outline of subjects according to the individual needs of their program and targeted service population. The suggested outline of subjects has been expanded beyond the minimal course competency requirements to provide an overview of a broad and comprehensive Home Health Aide program. In addition, before expanding program training and services beyond the minimum course competencies, it is important to verify with individual state nursing boards the invasive procedures that cannot be performed by anyone other than a licensed nurse. Depending on individual state laws, agencies will find the expanded list of subjects to be included in the training program helpful in determining and meeting community needs for maternal–child paraprofessional support.

The training program was designed to be used by the instructor in combination with relevant nursing textbooks. The author uses and recommends the latest editions of Lippincott–Raven nursing textbooks for nursing fundamentals, maternity, pediatrics, and the Lippincott *Manual of Nursing Practice*, all of which can be found in the bibliography. Any program offering maternal–child health services is incomplete without a basic reference library for its staff.

CONTENT AND DURATION OF TRAINING

POLICY:

A Home Health Aide training program must provide instruction in each of the subject areas covered in the following procedure section through classroom and supervised practical training totaling at least 75 hours. At least 16 hours of classroom time instruction must take place before beginning patient care through supervised practical training.

Supervised practical training is training in a laboratory or other setting in which the trainee demonstrates knowledge while performing tasks with an individual under the direct supervision of a registered nurse. Before the supervised practical training portion of the program begins, the Home Health Aide Classroom Orientation Form is to be completed by the qualified nursing instructor and entered into the Home Health Aide's personnel file.

As part of the documentation required to demonstrate compliance with the conditions for Home Health Aide services, the supervised practical training component of the Home Health Aide program must be documented on a form known as the Home Health Aide Supervised Practical Training Form. The supervised practical training must be evaluated and documented after observation of the aide's performance of a task with a patient. Tasks include reading and recording temperature, monitoring pulse and respiration, and performing appropriate and safe techniques of personal hygiene and grooming. Among the personal hygiene and grooming tasks that must be mastered are the bed bath; sponge, tub, and shower baths; shampoo in sink, tub, or bed; nail and skin care; oral hygiene; toileting and elimination; safe transfer techniques in ambulation; and normal range of motion and positioning.

The Home Health Aide Supervised Practical Training Form must be completed for each of these areas by the qualified nurse instructor. All subject areas in the home health agency program are evaluated through written examination, oral classroom participation, and/or after observation of a Home Health Aide with a patient. All observations are documented on the Home Health Aide Supervised Practical Training Form.

The Home Health Aide shall take a written examination prepared by the registered nurse instructor. This examination shall be graded on a numerical scale on which a grade above 70 shall be considered satisfactory and a grade below 70 shall be considered unsatisfactory. The Home Health Aide Supervised Practical Training Form, the Home Health Aide Orientation Form, and the Home Health Aide written examination will be entered into the personnel file of the Home Health Aide by the registered nurse instructor to demonstrate and document determination of appropriate Home Health Aide competency.

PURPOSE:

The training procedures are designed to assure provision of Home Health Aide services by appropriately qualified personnel.

PROCEDURE:

The individual being trained will complete at least 16 hours of classroom training prior to the beginning of the supervised practical training component of the program. Upon completion of the 16 hours of classroom training, the trainee will complete a program of at least 59 additional hours devoted to supervised practical training provided under the supervision of a qualified registered nurse. The total training will require 75 hours to complete.

Training will include the following subject areas.

1. Reading and recording temperature, pulse, and respiration
2. Appropriate and safe techniques in personal hygiene and grooming
    a. Bed bath
    b. Sponge, tub, or shower bath
    c. Shampoo: in sink, tub, or bed
    d. Nail and skin care
    e. Oral hygiene
    f. Toileting and elimination
    g. Safe transfer technique, ambulating, normal range of motion, and positioning must be evaluated after observation of performance of the tasks with a patient.

    Other subject matters requiring evaluation through written evaluation, oral examination, or after observation of the Home Health Aide with a patient include the following.

1. Communication skills
2. Observation, reporting, and documentation of patient status and care or service furnished
3. Basic infection control procedures
4. Basic elements and body functioning and changes in body functioning that must be reported to the aide supervisor
5. Maintenance of a clean, safe, and healthy environment
6. Recognition of emergencies and knowledge of emergency procedures
7. Physical, emotional, and developmental needs of and ways to work with the population served by the home health agency, including the need for respect for the patient, for his or her privacy, and for his or her property.
8. Adequate nutrition and fluid intake
9. Other tasks the home health agency may choose to have the Home Health Aide perform

    The supervising nurse is responsible for maintaining sufficient documentation to demonstrate that the requirements of these standards are met.

EVALUATION AND IN-SERVICE TRAINING

The Home Health Aide competency evaluation program and in-service training may be offered by any organization except a home health agency that has been determined to be out of compliance with one or more of the requirements of the Medicare conditions of participation within 24 months of the beginning of the training program.

POLICY: The home health agency will assure maintenance of all conditions of participation for Home Health Aide services to conduct competency evaluation and training of Home Health Aides.

PROCEDURE: The administrator on a semiannual basis will provide an opportunity for a written evaluation of the Home Health Aide program. This evaluation is based on the ability of the Home Health Aide services to meet all necessary requirements, standards, and conditions of participation. This documentation shall be kept by the administrator as separate administrative records and made available to appropriate agency evaluators.

QUALIFICATIONS FOR HOME HEALTH AIDE INSTRUCTORS

POLICY: The training of Home Health Aides and the supervision of Home Health Aides during the supervised practical portion of the training must be performed by or under the general supervision of a registered nurse who possesses a minimum of 2 years of nursing experience, with at least 1 year in the provision of Home Health Aide care, and has supervised Home Health Aide services for at least 6 months. Other individuals may be used to provide instruction under the supervision of the qualified registered nurse. The supervising nurse or a designated delegate of the agency shall meet minimum qualifications as an instructor for the training of Home Health Aides and the supervision of Home Health Aides during the supervised practical portion of the training.

PURPOSE: The requirements for the supervising nurse are designed to assure appropriate training of Home Health Aides by qualified professional individuals.

PROCEDURE: The administrator shall assure recruitment of a supervising nurse who meets the minimum qualifications for a Home Health Aide instructor, which include a minimum of 2 years of nursing experience, with at least 1 year in the provision of home care, and supervision of Home Health Aide services for at least 6 months.

The supervising nurse candidate must show evidence of work experience in the employment application completed for the agency and/or within his or her resume. The candidate must provide at least two written references that may be checked by the administrator to verify the candidate's possession of the minimum qualifications. Documentation of minimum qualifications as an instructor in the Home Health Aide training program will be entered into the personnel file of the individual to assure appropriate demonstration that the requirements of this standard have been met.

QUALIFICATIONS FOR PERFORMING COMPETENCY EVALUATIONS AND ONGOING IN-SERVICE TRAINING

POLICY: Competency evaluation must be performed by a registered nurse, and in-service training generally must be supervised by a registered nurse who possesses a minimum of 2 years in nursing experience, with at least 1 year in the provision of home health care, and who has supervised home health service for at least 6 months. The supervising nurse or qualified delegate will act as the Home Health Aide instructor and evaluator and must possess a minimum of 2 years of nursing experience providing home health care and must have supervised Home Health Aide services for at least 6 months.

PURPOSE: The requirements for competency evaluation and in-service training are designed to provide compliance with standards assuring appropriate Home Health Aide instruction and evaluation by qualified professional personnel.

PROCEDURE: Registered nurses participating as Home Health Aide evaluators and/or instructors will provide documentation to the agency of their minimum of 2 years of nursing experience, with at least 1 year providing home care and at least 6 months supervising Home Health Aide services. The agency will document this experience and complete the appropriate reference checks with former employers.

CONDUCTIVE TRAINING

POLICY: The Home Health Aide training program may be offered by any organization except a home health agency that has been determined to be out of compliance with one or more of the Federal Medicare requirements within the 24 months before the training program is to begin.

PURPOSE: The requirements of the Home Health Aide training program are designed to assure appropriate agency compliance with conditions of participation for Home Health Aide services.

PROCEDURE: The supervising nurse or qualified designee is responsible for the development, implementation, and administration/supervision of the Home Health Aide training program.

The supervising nurse and, if applicable, the qualified designee will maintain adequate continuing education to assure ongoing knowledge satisfying the requirements of the agency's Home Health Aide program. The supervising nurse or qualified designee shall maintain all Home Health Aide training program policies, procedures, and personnel files sufficient to document that the standards and Medicare conditions of participation for Home Health Aide training are met.

The supervising nurse shall assure performance of an annual review and evaluation of the Home Health Aide training program. The supervising nurse will make recommendations to the governing body through the administrator of the agency regarding recommended changes in the program based on the annual review and evaluation. Under the direction of the administrator, the supervising nurse will be responsible to the governing body to act upon any recommendations from the governing body or professional advisory committee. Any recommendations made should be based on the results of the annual program evaluation, and the supervising nurse will assure inclusion of these recommendations into the overall Home Health Aide training program.

DOCUMENTATION OF INITIAL TRAINING AND ONGOING IN-SERVICE EDUCATION FOR HOME HEALTH AIDES

POLICY: The home health agency must maintain sufficient documentation to demonstrate that the requirements of the Home Health Aide standards and Medicare conditions of participation are met.

PURPOSE: Appropriate documentation must demonstrate that personnel qualifications, training, and in-service training meet the conditions of participation for home health services.

PROCEDURE: The training of Home Health Aides and the supervision of Home Health Aides during the supervised practical portion of training must be performed by or under the general supervision of a registered nurse who possesses a minimum of 2 years of nursing experience, at least 1 year of which has been in home health care, and who has supervised Home Health Aide services for at least 6 months. Other individuals may be used to provide instruction under the supervision of the qualified registered nurse. The agency will maintain sufficient documentation that the requirements of this standard are met.

Policies and procedures of the Home Health Aide program will reflect the agency's intent to secure instructors with the best qualifications. Documentation demonstrating that the requirements of this standard are met will be furnished in the following ways.

1. The applicant will indicate his or her qualifications on the employment application and/or resume.
2. The administrator will obtain a signed reference release and will then verify the applicant's qualifications with former employers or with the agency supervisor.
3. These qualifications, as criteria for the position, will be documented as part of the job description for Home Health Aide instructors.
4. Depending on individual agency or individual state or local requirements, child abuse clearance and or criminal background check, although always desirable, may be required.

SUBJECT AREAS OF THE HOME HEALTH AIDE'S COMPETENCY EVALUATION

POLICY: The following are subject areas in which the Home Health Aide must demonstrate satisfactory competence, which in turn must be documented by the agency.

1. Communication skills.
2. Observation, reporting, and documentation of patient status and services furnished.
3. Reading and recording of temperature, pulse, and respiration.

4. Knowledge of and practice of basic infection control procedures.

5. Understanding of basic elements of body functioning and changes in body function that must be reported to the aide's supervisor.

6. Ability to maintain a clean, safe, and healthy environment.

7. Recognition of emergencies and knowledge of emergency procedures.

8. Awareness of the physical, emotional, and developmental needs of the population served by the home health agency, as well as the ways to work with this population. This includes the need for respect for the patient, for his or her privacy, and for his or her property.

9. Mastery of appropriate and safe techniques in personal hygiene, including the following skills.
   a. Bed bath
   b. Sponge, tub, or shower bath
   c. Shampoo: in sink, tub, or bed
   d. Nail and skin care
   e. Oral hygiene
   f. Toileting and elimination
   g. Safe transfer techniques and ambulation
   h. Normal range of motion and positioning
   i. Adequate nutrition and fluid intake
   j. Any other task that the home health agency may choose to have the Home Health Aide perform

DOCUMENTATION OF ANNUAL PERFORMANCE EVALUATION AND IN-SERVICE TRAINING

POLICY: Home Health Aides are required to have an annual performance evaluation and quarterly in-service training that must be documented by the agency.

PURPOSE: Annual performance evaluations and in-service training requirements demonstrate agency compliance in assuring that all personnel providing Home Health Aide services are determined to be competent and appropriately trained.

PROCEDURE: The completed Home Health Aide Performance Review Form will be signed by the Home Health Aide and the registered nurse providing the evaluation. Upon completion, the signed performance evaluation will be included as part of the Home Health Aide's personnel file.

The agency will maintain a written record of all in-service training in the Home Health Aide's personnel file and in a central agency location. The qualifications of the instructor must be included. Documentation of Home Health

Aide initial training, content and frequency of evaluations, and amount of in-service training will be completed through the following process.

Initial orientation and training will be documented through the Home Health Aide Classroom Orientation Form, the Home Health Aide Supervised Practical Training Form, and the Home Health Aide written examination. The content and frequency of evaluations and the amount of in-service training will be documented through the qualified nurse evaluator's completion of a performance review on the Home Health Aide Performance Review Form for each Home Health Aide no less frequently than every 12 months. Home Health Aide in-service training will be documented on the Home Health Aide In-Service Training Report. The Home Health Aide in-service training form will be entered into and become part of the Home Health Aide's personnel file.

OUTLINE OF SUGGESTED TOPICS FOR A HOME HEALTH AIDE TRAINING PROGRAM

Unit I: Introduction

1. Introduction
   An introduction to the program, to the role of the Home Health Aide, and to the rights of the patient
   a. Orientation to the organization
      1) Philosophy and goals
      2) History of organization
      3) Staff and administrative structure
   b. Role of the Home Health Aide
      1) Part of the home health care team
      2) Responsibilities
      3) Overview of duties
      4) Expectations and connection to organization
      5) Characteristics of Home Health Aides
   c. Overview of training program
      1) Schedule
      2) Responsibilities
      3) Certification process
2. Expected outcome
   Upon completion, the Home Health Aide will understand the following.
   a. Philosophy and goals of the organization
   b. Role of the Home Health Aide
   c. Extent of the training program

d. Home Health Aide's relationship to the organization

e. Patient rights, including the need for respect for the patient, for his or her right to privacy, and for his or her property

3. Content: Overview of training
The training program consists of 75 hours of instruction. Successful completion of the course includes attendance at classes; completion of all assigned work; satisfactory demonstration of procedures; satisfactory completion of written, verbal, and practical examinations; and a satisfactory review by the training instructor. A copy of the Patient Rights is enclosed within the medical record section of this manual for review.

4. Training activities
   a. Goal: The Home Health Aide will become familiar with the organization.
   b. Activities
      1) Review history of organization, philosophy, and goals.
      2) Discuss goals of home care.
      3) Review outline of Home Health Aide's duties.
      4) Have students list their ideas of the characteristics of a Home Health Aide and compare to summary.
      5) Review Patient Rights. (See Clinical Records.)

Unit II: Course Content

The Home Health Aide training program will consist of 75 hours of basic training. The Home Health Aide will complete verbal, written, and practical examinations and will receive a certificate after satisfactory completion of the course and examinations.

A significant part of the training will be devoted to care of the pregnant woman, the high-risk infant, the normal neonate, the infant, and the child. The training will be based on the family and how the events of the illness, delivery, or maternal complications affect the family as a unit.

The program content should be targeted by the instructor to address the individual needs of the organization. The learning modules offer the instructor a maternal–child health core course that should be used in conjunction with the suggested nursing textbooks to present the most current available disease-specific information.

1. Introduction
Suggested teaching materials: Individual organization philosophy and goals material; personnel section of this manual.
   a. Introduction to the organization
      1) Philosophy and goals
      2) Role of the Home Health Aide
      3) Expectations of the organization
   b. Self-care
   Suggested teaching materials: Individual organization personnel policies; Module 1 for student and instructor
      1) Maintaining good physical health
      2) Maintaining good emotional health and handling stress

c. Time and energy management
Suggested teaching materials: Modules 1 and 2 for student and instructor

1) Conserving time and energy
2) Use of resources
3) Body mechanics (basic prevention of injuries)

2. Working with people
Suggested teaching materials: Modules 1, 2, and 4 for student and instructor

a. Basic human needs and the family

1) Importance of the family in society
2) Basic needs and unmet needs
3) Reaction of individuals/family to illness
4) Role of Home Health Aide in meeting needs

b. Developmental process of parenting
Suggested teaching materials: Modules 1, 5, and 6 for student and instructor

1) Normal process of pregnancy, labor, and delivery.
2) Problems of interrupted development.
3) Development of parenting roles

c. Communications
Suggested teaching materials: Modules 1 and 4 for student and instructor

1) Methods, types, and levels
2) Techniques of listening
3) Communication with children

3. Personal care and procedures
Suggested teaching materials: Modules 5 and 6 for student and instructor; recommended nursing textbooks for instructor

a. Care of the patient on bedrest

1) Personal hygiene
2) Turning, positioning, and exercising
3) Emotional support

b. Vital signs

1) Normals
2) Techniques
3) Variations

c. Procedures

1) Enemas
2) Hot and cold applications
3) Compresses
4) Ace bandages, slings, and dressings

5) Review of clean/sterile technique
6) Irrigation of wounds, dressing
7) Observations
8) Intake and output
9) Collecting specimens
10) Self-administered medications
11) Assisting with ambulation
12) Range of motion
13) Catheter care

d. Infection control
Suggested teaching materials: Module 3 for student and instructor

1) Review of causes of infection
2) Organisms and their growth
3) Handwashing
4) Disposal of waste
5) Maintaining a clean environment
6) Prevention of infection

4. Care of the pregnant woman
Suggested teaching materials: Module 6 for student and instructor; recommended nursing textbooks for instructor

a. Prenatal care
b. Normal discomforts of pregnancy
   1) Etiology
   2) Comfort measures
c. Pregnancy complications
d. Warning signs in pregnancy
e. Premature labor versus term labor
f. Pregnancy bedrest

5. Newborn care
Suggested teaching materials: Module 5 for student and instructor; recommended nursing text for instructor

a. Normal newborn
   1) Characteristics
   2) Physical care
   3) Feeding/nutrition, breastfeeding
   4) Variations of normal
   5) Handling normal infant problems
   6) Immunizations
   7) Developmental needs

8) Special care

b. Newborn with problems
Suggested teaching materials: Module 5 for student and instructor; recommended nursing textbooks for instructor

1) Etiology
2) Problems common to the high-risk infant
3) Differences in care needs
4) Feeding and gastrointestinal problems
5) Respiratory problems
6) Growth and development problems
7) Cardiac problems
8) Renal problems
9) Special procedures
    (a) Oro-nasogastric feedings
    (b) Apnea monitor
    (c) Ostomies
    (d) Oxygen
10) Prematurity
    (a) Etiology
    (b) Characteristics
    (c) Physical needs
    (d) Developmental needs
    (e) Supporting parents
    (f) Long-term problems

c. Developmental needs
Suggested teaching materials: Modules 1, 5, and 6 for student and instructor; recommended nursing textbooks for instructor

1) Play
2) Stimulation
3) Identifying delays
4) Teaching parents
5) Norms of growth and development
6) Safety

d. Care needs

1) Fluids/hydration
2) Medication
3) Physical care
    (a) Managing fever

(b) Handling rashes

(c) Personal hygiene

4) Special procedures

(a) Croupette

(b) Oxygen

(c) Gastrostomy feeding

(d) Continuous night feeding

(e) Postural drainage

(f) Mini-nebulizer

(g) Range of motion, other physical therapy

(h) Intravenous therapy

e. Managing acute illness

1) Respiratory disease

2) Gastrointestinal disease

3) Infection

4) Communicable illness

f. Managing chronic illness

1) Respiratory compromise

2) Asthma

3) Cancer

4) Diabetes

5) Cerebral palsy

6) Mental retardation

7) Care needs

8) Procedures

9) Developmental needs and care

10) Support of family

11) The dying child

6. Nutrition
Suggested teaching materials: Modules 2, 3, 5, and 6 for student and instructor; recommended nursing textbooks for instructor

a. Normal diet

b. Special diets

c. Meal preparation and serving (bottle preparation)

7. Documentation
Suggested teaching materials: Clinical Records section of this manual for student and instructor; personnel and training forms in this manual for student and instructor

   a. Proper recording methods
   b. Information necessary to record
   c. Organization records
   d. Confidentiality (medical records and phone)

8. Emergency care
   Suggested teaching materials: Module 1 for student and instructor; parent educational section of this manual for student and instructor

ROLE OF THE NURSE IN SUPERVISING THE HOME HEALTH AIDE

The Home Health Aide is a part of the entire home health care team and needs and wants the support, supervision, and assistance of the nurse. Home Health Aides are trained to understand the spectrum of home care and their own responsibilities. They should be trained to conduct an environmental and family assessment to begin planning their own work. They will be expected to plan the work they will do for each case, sometimes on a daily basis, sometimes on a weekly basis. The Home Health Aide will expect the nurse to review the care plan with him or her and to make suggestions. The Home Health Aides will be looking to the nurse for guidance, in planning, in what to observe the patient for, and in how to perform procedures and treatments.

As part of the routine report, please give the Home Health Aide the courtesy of looking thoroughly over the notes he or she has made and discussing appropriate alterations. Give your support by listening to and recording the concerns of the Home Health Aide and by offering suggestions for handling difficult situations. Make a note of any procedures that are new to him or her and record the quality of care in that area. Periodically the nurse will be asked to complete case reviews or performance reviews.

The Home Health Aide's responsibilities might be divided into several categories for convenience of planning and evaluation. These include the following areas.

1. Household and family assessment for planning

2. Household management
   a. Meal preparation
   b. Maintaining family routines
   c. Cleaning
   d. Laundry

3. Personal care of patient

4. Psychosocial support
   a. Emotional support of patient or family members
   b. Referral to nurse for resources
   c. Identification of serious social problems
   d. Companionship
   e. Intake and output

f. Range of motion and other physical therapy activities
g. Supervision of certain procedures
h. Observation of the patient for untoward signs and for progress

5. Child care
   a. Babysitting of well children
   b. Care of newborn

Each Home Health Aide will keep progress notes. On the form for these notes there is a column for the supervising nurse to initial and/or to comment. Please record comments freely.

The supervising nurse should be available to the Home Health Aide at any time for a problem, assistance, or support.

CONTENT AND AMOUNT OF IN-SERVICE TRAINING

The Home Health Aide must receive at least 3 hours of in-service training per calendar quarter. In-service training may be furnished while the aide is furnishing care to the patient.

POLICY: The supervising nurse shall be responsible to plan at least 3 hours of training per quarter for the Home Health Aide. The supervising nurse shall have the authority to require all Home Health Aides to attend these in-service training sessions.

PURPOSE: In-service training is provided to assure compliance with standards for conditions of participation regarding in-service training.

PROCEDURE: A supervising nurse who also meets the qualifications for a Home Health Aide instructor shall plan at least 3 hours of in-service training per calendar quarter as part of the Home Health Aide services program.

The supervising nurse will prepare the in-service training or recruit community professionals to provide training that will assist the Home Health Aide in the further understanding of patient and family needs. The supervising nurse shall plan these in-service training sessions on an annual basis to be conducted quarterly. Planning the in-service training sessions for the entire year at once makes it easier to accommodate the scheduling of Home Health Aide time. In this manner, attendance will be facilitated by planning for appropriate patient coverage prior to the training session if the time conflicts with that of direct patient care.

The supervising nurse shall document each Home Health Aide's participation in at least 3 hours of in-service training per calendar year on the Home Health Aide in-service training form. This shall become part of the Home Health Aide personnel file, to document that the Home Health Aide training requirements have been met.

CHAPTER 3

Home Health Aide Training Modules

Chapter 3 contains a core course for paraprofessionals in providing care to the maternal–child population. The learning modules included address areas of child and household safety, household management, communication, care of the pregnant and postpartum woman, and care of the newborn. Providers can best use the modules by distributing them to trainees for study and reference. The modules offer to-the-point information that must be known by the Home Health Aide before providing care without direct supervision of a nurse. It is recommended that each trainee receive his or her own copy of these modules. In addition, providers can use this format to develop advanced training modules based on the needs of the community and allowable paraprofessional services according to the individual state nursing board.

MODULE 1: SAFETY

Safety Precautions

This section covers the safety precautions the Family-Centered Home Health Aide should use to protect the family and himself or herself in the home. Upon completion of this unit, the learner should be prepared to accomplish the following.

1. Describe the elements of practicing electrical safety.
   a. Do not place electrical cords where they will be tripped over or get excessive wear (under rugs, through doorways, etc.).
   b. Keep electrical cords away from heat and water.
   c. Do not pull the cord to disconnect; rather, pull the plug itself. Avoid kinking, twisting, binding, or crushing the cord.
   d. Inspect cords for wear, especially at connections; do not use a cord that has a break exposing wires.
   e. Never turn on an appliance when standing on a wet floor, and do not put any electrical parts in water.
   f. Do not touch plumbing or a metal object and an appliance at the same time.
   g. Follow manufacturers' instructions for operation and care.
   h. Disconnect any appliance that sparks or stalls.
   i. Keep combustible materials (clothing, curtains, paper, etc.) away from lamps or heating devices.
   j. Always disconnect appliances before cleaning.
   k. Never touch broken outside wires. Notify mother or other adult member of household to call police and electric company. Warn others to keep away.
   l. Never "play" electrician.
   m. Always notify family of any actions you take and your reasons for taking them.
2. Identify damage that may occur to the body in the event of an electrical shock.
   a. Chest muscles contract, interfering with breathing.
   b. Nerve center paralysis can result in inability to breathe.
   c. Normal heart rhythm interrupted, which can cause blood circulation to stop.
   d. Hemorrhages and destruction of tissue, nerves, and/or muscle can occur.
3. Identify safety measures to protect oneself while cooking.
   a. Do not reach over an open flame with arm.
   b. Do not cook wearing garments with large, loose sleeves. Roll sleeves up. Most severe burns are caused by clothing that has caught fire.
   c. Do not mix hot oil with water. This can cause a hot oil burn.
   d. Turn off flame before adding any food to hot oil to prevent flame from shooting up and "tracking" the oil splatter. Flame should be adjusted appropriately after food is in pan.

e. Watch for children "underfoot" while carrying trays with hot liquids or foods to avoid tripping and causing a burn or injury.

f. Check oven and stove to be sure they are off when finished cooking.

4. Identify first aid actions in case of a burn.

   a. Stop burning process to prevent further tissue destruction; remove from the source of injury.

   b. When clothes catch fire, victim should fall to floor or ground and roll in carpet or blanket if available; otherwise, ***stop***, ***drop***, ***roll***, and beat out flames with anything available.

      1) Running causes flames to spread.

      2) Standing still would force victim to breathe flames and smoke and could cause hair to be ignited.

   c. Remove clothing only if smoldering or hot or in the case of a scald burn (clothing holds heat).

   d. Initiate immediate care of victim.

      1) Small areas

         (a) Immerse burned areas in cool water for 10 minutes or apply cool water compresses. This limits tissue destruction and helps prevent further complications.

         (b) Notify family of situation.

         (c) Contact Home Care Supervisor for instructions.

         (d) Do not apply any ointments to area.

      2) Large, exposed areas

         (a) Stop burning process, allow wound to cool.

         (b) Call out for family member and have someone contact police, fire, or emergency squad.

         (c) Have member of family contact Home Care Supervisor if you are burned.

         (d) If a family member is the burn victim, contact Home Care Supervisor yourself when the emergency is under control.

      3) Chemical burns

         (a) Irrigate with large quantities of running water (except for burns caused by phosphorus, in which case instructions should be noted on package contents).

         (b) Have someone call police, fire, or emergency squad.

         (c) Cover with loosely applied clean cloth.

         (d) Contact Home Care Supervisor.

      4) Chemical burns of eye

         (a) Have someone in household call police, fire, or emergency squad.

         (b) Remove contact lenses or have person remove them.

         (c) Hold eye directly under running water with eyelids pulled back until emergency team arrives.

         (d) Contact Home Care Supervisor.

5) Electrical burns

If victim is in contact with live, indoor, low-voltage electricity:

(a) Shut off power if possible (pull plug, turn off switch).

(b) If shutting off power is not possible, free victim (use dry rope, stick, wooden plank, etc.). Be sure that your hands are dry and that you are on a dry surface.

(c) Have someone in the household contact the police, fire, or emergency squad.

(d) Establish an airway and, ***if indicated, initiate CPR—if you are certified***.

(e) Keep victim warm and keep head lower than feet unless head injury is possibly involved.

(f) Give detailed report to medical transport team.

(g) Contact Home Care Supervisor.

If victim is in contact with live ***outdoor*** wire, the only safe procedure is to call the utility company and allow them to turn off the power.

e. Never use water to extinguish an electrical fire.

1) Water is an electrical conductor—you will be electrocuted.

2) Extinguish electrical fire with dry chemical extinguisher or dry chemical only.

5. Identify 10 elements contributing to poor safety attitudes.

a. Cynicism: "That safety stuff is junk."

b. Fatalism: "Well, accidents do happen."

c. Laziness: "It's too much work."

d. Temper: "I'll do it my way."

e. Forgetfulness: "I thought to. . . . but. . . . "

f. Carelessness: "I was paying attention to something else."

g. Ignorance: "I didn't know it was poison."

h. Overconfidence: "Things like that never happen to me."

i. Recklessness: "It's not that bad."

j. Showing off: "Look at what I can do."

6. Identify your personal responsibilities in on-the-job safety.

a. Come to work relaxed. Fatigue is a frequent factor in the cause of accidents.

b. Know and follow the rules of safety and familiarize yourself with the use of equipment in the house.

c. Know what to do in case of an emergency.

7. Identify actions that will prevent injury resulting from moving things.

a. Lifting

1) Look at the item to be moved. Make sure it is not too bulky or heavy.

2) Stand close to the object and spread feet apart for balance. Make sure your footing feels secure.

3) Bend your knees and keep your back straight.

4) Grasp the object with a good grip and keep it close to your body.

5) Lift slowly, using thigh and calf muscles. Keep your back straight and avoid quick motions.

b. Carrying

1) Keep the object close to your body.

2) Hold it securely with both hands.

3) Avoid twisting your body; change direction by moving your feet.

4) Do not change your handgrip while carrying; place the item back down and start again if your grip is failing.

5) Face the spot where you are putting the item down.

c. Pushing and pulling

1) Get a good grip on the object to be moved.

2) Keep your back straight.

3) Brace your feet and use your thigh and calf muscles.

4) Bend your knees for best use of body weight.

8. Identify safety actions to be taken in preventing accidental falls.

a. Pick up everything spilled or dropped on the floor.

b. Pull wheeled vehicles through doorways so you can see where you are going.

c. Use a stepladder for out-of-reach things; chairs, stools, etc. lead to accidents.

d. Watch your step. Watch for toddlers underfoot and do not read while walking. Do not obstruct your vision with high loads.

e. Use handrails when going up and down steps.

f. Walk at a safe speed.

g. Watch for pantlegs that are too long and shoelaces that may come untied.

h. Watch for items on or across floors that contribute to hazardous walking.

i. Avoid groping in dark closets.

j. Wear sensible shoes—no clogs or sandals permitted on the job.

k. Watch for items left on stairs, such as toys, etc.

l. Identify measures to help prevent accidental cuts and punctures.

1) Watch for loose knives in drawers when reaching inside. Any sharp items to be disposed of should be carefully wrapped in paper.

2) Do not reach into wastebaskets while emptying.

3) Use scoops or gloves when handling chemicals, detergents, or cleaning agents.

4) Do not try to catch a sharp item that falls. Move out of the way. Sweep up after it is on the ground.

5) Promptly sweep up broken glass and keep children out of the area. Damp mop to be sure all glass splinters are picked up. Instruct children to wear shoes.

6) Be careful to avoid catching fingers in drawers.

9. Identify elements in prevention of machinery accidents.
    a. Always request instruction manual or owner's instructions prior to use.
    b. Never leave machines plugged in and unattended (e.g., mixers, can openers, food processors, etc.).
    c. Watch your clothing around moving parts.
    d. If you are uncomfortable with a particular machine, inform the client that you will be unable to use it.

10. Identify the three elements necessary to produce a fire.
    a. Air
    b. Heat
    c. Fuel

11. Identify emergency procedures in case of a fire.
    a. Yell "FIRE" loud enough for the entire household to hear.
    b. Use a fire extinguisher if easily available and the flame is very small.
    c. Quickly check for which class of fire the extinguisher is designed.
        1) Class A: paper, wood, rags, cardboard
        2) Class B: flammable liquids
        3) Class C: all electrical equipment

        An ABC extinguisher can be used for all types of fires.
    d. Pull pin located in the head of the extinguisher.
    e. Use the fire extinguisher like a broom. Sweep from side to side at base of fire.
    f. If a fire extinguisher is not easily available, or if the fire is too large, or if the fire cannot be contained by an extinguisher, ***get the family and yourself out of the house quickly!***
    g. Call the fire department after the entire household has been evacuated.

Safety-Promoting Activities

This section covers activities the Family-Centered Home Health Aide can undertake to protect and provide for the safety of the childbearing family in their home. Upon completion of this unit, the learner should be prepared to accomplish the following.

1. List six safety measures for bathing the infant.
    a. Check water temperature with elbow, making sure water is only warm, not hot, to avoid scalding.
    b. Keep water faucets off during bath to avoid scalding or splashing in face.
    c. Never leave the baby alone in the bath for any reason. It takes only seconds to drown.
    d. Keep one hand on the baby at all times during the bath to prevent him or her from slipping.

e. Wrap the baby up and take him or her with you if something else requires your immediate attention.

f. Organize all the items you will need before the bath to prevent having to take the baby out of the bath and causing a chill.

2. List 13 actions you should take to protect the infant/toddler from accidental injury.

   a. Keep pins and other sharp objects such as scissors and knives out of the baby's reach. Instruct parents to use only diaper pins with plastic shields to prevent accidental cuts, punctures, or serious injury.

   b. Pick up buttons, beads, hairpins, and any other small items on the floor. This prevents accidental swallowing and/or choking. A baby can find the smallest item on the cleanest floor.

   c. If not in place, ask parents if they have safety plugs or outlet covers. Young fingers can find their way into a socket easily.

   d. When possible, remove easily overturned lamps, electric cords, and sharp-edged furniture. Always keep fans out of fingers' reach to prevent accidental injury.

   e. Fold parts of the tablecloth hanging in the child's reach up onto the table, because one quick pull may spill everything on the table on top of the baby. This prevents accidental injury.

   f. Always keep pot handles turned to the inside of the stove and use back burners whenever possible, because young babies will try to stand up against the range and pull pots over; toddlers and young children may be quick to do the same. This prevents accidental burns.

   g. Always make sure the siderails of the crib are up before leaving the baby, to prevent accidental falls.

   h. Always keep one hand on the baby while on the changing table, to prevent accidental falls.

   i. Never leave the baby unattended anywhere in the house. If necessary, place the baby in a playpen or crib with the sides up to prevent accidental injury.

   j. If available, place a gate across stairways. Test the gate by pushing against it to make sure it is firm. If a gate is unavailable, use other household items to block stairs safely to prevent an accidental fall down the steps.

   k. Always lock doors that lead to stairways, porches, driveways, yards, storage, and any other dangerous area to prevent child from wandering into the area.

   l. Lock windows and/or screens on all windows above the first floor to prevent accidental falls.

   m. Never leave the iron on the ironing board even if it is unplugged, because a young child may knock it over. An iron is very heavy and has a sharp pointed edge. Safe handling will prevent burns, concussion, and/or serious cuts.

3. List 11 items that can be the cause of infant smothering, strangulation, and/or suffocation. Plastic bags, long toy telephone cords, harnesses, soft pillows, Venetian blind cords (watch cribs and playpens next to windows), balloons, small objects, large pieces of food, necklaces, pacifier cords, pieces of plants (which can also cause poisoning).

4. List nine ways to prevent accidental burns.

   a. Place guards in front of open heaters, fireplaces, steam radiators, and floor furnaces.

b. Keep hot liquids, hot foods, and electric cords of irons, toasters, and coffeepots out of reach. Pot handles should be turned in. Use back burners.

c. Always test foods and bottles for temperature before serving.

d. Keep matches and/or cigarette lighters locked up or on your person.

e. Never leave young children or babies alone in the kitchen.

f. Do not allow young children to turn on hot water faucets.

g. Do not allow young children to step into a bath unless you have tested the water temperature.

h. Place electric cords or electric extension cords loosely behind furniture; young children may chew on these, especially when teething.

i. Provide ashtrays to smoking guests of the clients, making sure all cigarettes are dead when the guests leave.

5. List the safety concerns in the child's play area.

   a. The play area should be fenced in; if not, you should remain outside with the children; a child younger than 3 years old should not be in any type of yard alone.

   b. Lock up all matches, furniture polish, cleaning agents (paying special attention to lye, detergents, cleansers, toilet bowl cleaners, and drain cleaners), and medications.

   c. Provide unbreakable toys with no small removable parts for the child under 3; watch a child under 3 years of age playing with older siblings' toys.

   d. Provide constant supervision.

   e. Do not allow children in a swimming pool without supervision, explaining to the parent that you must either watch children in the pool or do other items needed in the household.

6. Identify examples of dangerous and safe toys by age group.

   a. Up to 2 years old

      1) Dangerous toys

         (a) Sponge or Nerf-type items that a child may bite.

         (b) Toys that are small enough to swallow.

         (c) Toys with small removable parts.

         (d) Stuffed animals or dolls with glass or button eyes, attachments, or hair that can be pulled out and eaten.

      2) Safe toys

         (a) Sturdy rattles (watch inside parts)

         (b) Large beads on strong cord

         (c) Large balls (soft, not Nerf-type balls)

         (d) Large one-piece bath toys and cups

         (e) Containers and objects for "putting into and emptying" play

         (f) Large and medium boxes

         (g) Push and pull toys

(h) Toys to ride, pushing with feet
(i) Rubber or cloth dolls with no small removable parts or hair
(j) Plastic dishpans for water, bubbles, or sand
(k) Pots, pans, and spoons

b. 2 to 3 years old
  1) Dangerous toys
    (a) Toys with sharp edges
    (b) Objects with small removable parts
    (c) Poisonous or lead paint
    (d) Marbles, jacks, beads, and coins
    (e) Flammable toys
    (f) Liquid crayon
    (g) Poorly balanced riding toys
  2) Safe toys
    (a) Floor trains, cars, and boats (nonelectrical)
    (b) Large peg boards
    (c) Wooden animals
    (d) Large crayons (only those labeled nontoxic)
    (e) Wooden puzzles with large pieces (6 to 10 pieces)
    (f) Clothes for dress-up
    (g) Big wheeled toys to ride
    (h) Balls, books, and large blocks
    (i) Music (child must not use record player alone)

c. 3 to 6 years old
  1) Dangerous toys
    (a) Sharp or cutting toys
    (b) Flammable costumes
    (c) Electrical toys
    (d) Shooting games and guns (a danger to eyes)
    (e) Poisonous paint sets
    (f) Poorly balanced trikes, bikes, wagons, and ride-on toys
    (g) Cement-type glue or Crazy Glue
  2) Safe toys
    (a) Easel and nontoxic washable paints and paint books
    (b) Basins, sponges, and soap for bubbles or dishwashing
    (c) Nontoxic bubbles for blowing
    (d) Nonelectric trains

(e) Blocks

(f) Dolls and equipment

(g) Action figures

(h) Blackboards and dustless chalk

(i) Modeling clay

(j) Games including Picture Lotto, Mousetrap, Candyland, Chutes and Ladders, and Lego. Look on the side of the box for appropriate age groups.

d. 6 to 12 years old

1) Dangerous toys

(a) Nonapproved electrical toys. Check toys to be sure they bear the UL (Underwriter's Laboratory) label. Check cords for patency.

(b) Sharp tools

(c) Poorly made sports equipment

(d) Shooting toys

(e) Bicycles that are either poorly balanced or have parts in need of repair

(f) Cement-type glue or Crazy Glue

2) Safe toys

(a) Video games (supervise electrical set-up)

(b) Hobby kits (instruct in use of glue)

(c) Crafts, games (such as checkers), crayons, construction sets, clay, and washable finger paints

(d) Tape recorders and record players (check cords)

Toys handled by the wrong age group can be very dangerous. Toys that are safe for the 6-year-old may be dangerous to the toddling sibling, for example. Have older children play with their toys, which may be unsafe for the younger ones, in an area inaccessible to younger siblings. Have older children pick up toys immediately after play to prevent accidents. You can make a game of this to encourage compliance.

7. Identify foods that may cause choking in the young child (infant to 2 years).
   a. Small pieces of zwieback toast or baby cookie. Supervise the child while eating. Distract the child and take away the toast or cookie while the pieces are still too large to fit entirely into the mouth.
   b. Small vegetables. Be sure to question parents as to what vegetables the child eats and how they are prepared (pureed, chopped, cut up, etc.).
   c. Uncooked spaghetti, rice, and beans
   d. Any small pieces of food the child may inhale or choke on because of immature chewing patterns
8. Identify the basics of traffic safety. If parents have given a child over 3 permission to play outside, take the following actions.
   a. Instruct the child to play out of the street and driveway.

b. Instruct the child to play with balls in the yard away from the street. Tell the child to come and get you if the ball should go into street, and emphasize that a new ball can be obtained if something happens to the one in use.

c. Question the parents as to the child's ability to play outside alone. If the parents give permission, be sure to check the child's activity every 15 minutes.

9. State the number of children poisoned annually and describe actions that can be taken to prevent accidental poisonings. List those agents commonly responsible for childhood poisonings.

   a. Poisoning is one of the most common childhood emergencies. Each year more than 500,000 children are poisoned. Some of these children die because poisoning is one of the most difficult emergencies to treat.

   b. Keep medicines, cleaning agents, and poisons out of sight and out of reach in a locked cabinet.

   c. Protect children from exposure to lead-based paint. Watch for paint chips, especially along windowsills and woodwork.

   d. Check household and outside areas for exposed medicines, cleaning agents, poisons, gasoline, kerosene, paint products, insecticides, and vitamins with iron. Remove these items from sight and reach. Ask the parents where items may be locked away. Plants may also be a source of poisoning. Instruct parents concerning the reasons for moving plants out of children's reach.

   e. Keep cleaning agents in hand when using them and locked up when not in use.

   f. The following are common sources of poisoning.

      1) Alcohol (Be careful about where the alcohol is kept for care of umbilical cord.)
      2) Aspirin, even baby aspirin
      3) Ammonia
      4) Bleaches
      5) Cosmetics (nail polish and polish removers, perm and hair color solutions)
      6) Detergents
      7) Fertilizers
      8) All medicines (including aspirin and other analgesics, iron pills, vitamins, cold medicines, tranquilizers, pills for pets, and children's vitamins)
      9) Furniture polishes and oils
      10) Kerosene, gasoline, lighter fluid, and all other petroleum-based products
      11) Moth balls
      12) Lye and other caustics (toilet and drain cleaners)
      13) Paint removers, thinners, and paints themselves; turpentine and household cleaners
      14) Pesticides (any insect control substance) and weed killers
      15) Plants
      16) If any items are in question, lock them up.

10. Identify eight emergency protocols in case of poisoning or suspected poisoning of a child.

    a. Inform the parent(s).

b. Try to identify what substance was swallowed and how much was taken.

c. Immediately call the Poison Control Center for advice about first aid treatment of the victim.

d. Follow the advice from the Poison Control Center. Enlist assistance from the parents or neighbors if necessary.

e. If the child is to be transported to a medical center, call 911 (or the local emergency number), the local police, or an ambulance service in the family's county. A relative should accompany the child to the hospital. Remain with other children if necessary.

f. Send container from which the child obtained the poison with the medical team. Document for them the time of ingestion, how much poison is thought to have originally been in the container (e.g., number of pills), instructions from Poison Control, and what measures were carried out.

g. Vomiting should not be induced in the following cases.

   1) If corrosive material such as lye or a strong acid has been swallowed

   2) If the child is drowsy, unconscious, or convulsive

h. After emergency procedures have been followed, contact the Home Care Supervisor as soon as possible.

11. Identify emergency protocols for the infant or child who is choking.

   a. The American Red Cross and the American Heart Association offer CPR classes. All home care personnel must take one of these programs within the first 3 months of employment and must be recertified annually. No one is qualified to render CPR to any client or client's infant or child under any conditions unless they are certified by the American Red Cross or the American Heart Association.

   b. If infant or child is choking, do nothing for 5 to 10 seconds.

      1) DO's

         (a) Wait for a cough.

         (b) Call for parent(s)—yell if necessary.

         (c) Hold the infant or child as illustrated by the instructor.

         (d) Have someone in the household dial 911 (or the local emergency number) immediately to summon the police, fire, or rescue squad, reminding the caller to state the emergency and give the address as calmly and clearly as possible.

         (e) Open the mouth and very gently try to remove the object.

         (f) If you are unsuccessful in removing the object, slap the infant or child firmly three or four times between the shoulder blades with the heel of your hand.

         (g) If the child is still choking after 1 minute, begin mouth to mouth resuscitation.

      2) DO NOT's

         (a) Jab your finger into the child's mouth.

         (b) Pull neck backward.

         (c) ***Do not panic!!***

   c. If the infant or child stops breathing and looks blue, begin mouth to mouth resuscitation.

1) Call out for someone in the household.
2) Have someone in the household dial 911 (or the local emergency number) immediately to summon the police, fire, or rescue squad, reminding the caller to state the emergency and give the address as calmly and clearly as possible.
3) Place the child on his or her back on top of a firm surface.
4) Tilt the child's head back slightly with the chin up (as demonstrated by the instructor, noting the difference in angle between a young infant and a child).
5) Cover the child's mouth and nose tightly with your mouth, allowing no breaks for air to escape.
6) Blow gently until chest moves. (Note that an infant requires less force than a child when blowing, so initiate resuscitation as "puffs.")
7) Remove your mouth and let the child's lungs empty.
8) Take a quick breath yourself.
9) Repeat at a rate of about 20 times per minute for a child or 30 times per minute for an infant.

d. If the chest does not move, very quickly check the position of the head, then try again. If there is still no movement, hold the child upside down and slap firmly between the shoulders. Check the mouth for blockage, but do not allow fingers to enter throat. Try again. ***Do not stop.*** If the heart has stopped and you are CPR-certified, begin CPR.

12. Identify the signs, symptoms, and actions to be taken in the event of infant breathing difficulties.

a. Signs and symptoms
1) Bluish color surrounding mouth and lips
2) Flaring of the nostrils with each breath
3) On breathing in and out, noise like a crow, wheezing, or grunt
4) Respiratory rate above 60 without excitement

b. Actions
1) Bring signs and symptoms to the attention of the parent(s).
2) Instruct the parent(s) to contact the pediatrician for instructions.
3) Assist parent(s) with any preparations for infant's physician visit.
4) Contact Home Care Supervisor.

13. Identify signs and symptoms of abdominal pain in the infant and specific emergency situations related to abdominal pain.

a. The abdomen feels tense, the legs are drawn up, and/or the fists are tightly clenched.
b. Occurs usually in late afternoon or evening.
c. Occurs in breast- or bottle-fed infants.
d. Instruct the parent(s) to contact the doctor immediately if the infant experiences any of the following symptoms.
1) Waves of pain
2) Straining and screaming

3) Looks pale and sweaty
4) Vomits yellowish green material
5) Vomits forcefully a distance of 1 to 2 feet after feeding and is still hungry
6) Has a reddish, jelly-like bowel movement
7) Has bloody bowel movements

14. Identify signs, symptoms, and actions to be taken when confronted by a convulsive infant, child, or adult.
    a. Signs and symptoms
        1) Body stiffens
        2) Eyes roll back into head
        3) Jerking movements of one or both sides of the body
        4) No response when name called
    b. Actions
        1) Call out for someone in the household.
        2) Have someone in the household contact the police, fire, or emergency squad by dialing 911 (or the local emergency number).
        3) Place victim on his or her left side or, if impossible, turn head to left side. This is important because the victim may vomit and breathe vomitus into the lungs.
        4) If breathing stops, gently check to be sure the airway is open and begin mouth to mouth resuscitation.

15. Identify actions to be taken in case of head injury to a child.
    a. Inform the parent(s) of the situation and have him or her notify the physician for further instructions.
    b. If the physician does not require the child to have a medical evaluation, continue to observe the child for problems that require an immediate return call to the physician.
        1) Nausea
        2) Vomiting
        3) Ataxia (walking off balance)
        4) Slurring of speech
        5) Occasional comment about blurred vision
        6) Sudden sleepiness

16. Identify actions to be taken in case of burns or scalds. If someone has been burned, take immediate steps to relieve the pain and prevent infection. If necessary, call emergency help as soon as possible. Burns are treated according to their severity.
    a. Degrees of burns
        1) First degree burns: outer skin is reddened and slightly swollen
        2) Second degree burns: under skin is also red and has blisters
        3) Third degree burns: skin is destroyed (white or charred appearance)

b. Treatment of burns

1) Minor burns: first degree

(a) To reduce pain, run cold water over the burn, then immerse the burned area in a container of cold water or apply cold towels frequently.

(b) Cover with sterile gauze or a clean bandage to prevent infection.

(c) If the burned area is fairly large, have someone in the household contact the physician.

(d) Notify Home Care Supervisor.

2) Major burns: second degree

(a) Have someone in the household contact the physician or police, fire, or emergency squad.

(b) Immerse the burned part in cold water or apply recently laundered cloths that have been dipped in cold water.

(c) Dry and cover with sterile gauze or a clean cloth.

(d) If an arm or leg has been burned, raise it so that it is higher than the victim's heart.

(e) Do not break blisters. Do not use cotton or any material with a loose fiber as a dressing. Do not apply any type of ointment or medication.

(f) Notify Home Care Supervisor.

3) Major burns: third degree

(a) Have someone in the household contact the police, fire, or emergency squad.

(b) Remove or cut away clothing from the burned area. If clothing sticks to the burn, do not pull it loose. Cut around the burned area.

(c) Watch for respiration problems. Use rescue breathing, if necessary.

(d) Apply a cold cloth to the face, hands, or feet, but do not immerse the burned area or apply cold packs to a large burned area because these actions may cause greater shock.

(e) Do not apply any medications.

(f) Follow any instructions given by the emergency team.

(g) Notify Home Care Supervisor.

4) Chemical burns

(a) Have someone in the household contact the police, fire, or emergency squad.

(b) Wash away the chemical with large quantities of water. Use a shower or hose while removing the victim's clothing. Wash away chemical completely. Do not use a neutralizing agent (such as soap); water is more effective. Then remove clothing, taking care not to tear the skin, which may adhere to the cloth.

(c) Cover the burned area with the cleanest available material.

(d) Notify Home Care Supervisor.

5) Eye burns

(a) If the victim is wearing contact lenses, have him or her remove them at once.

(b) Hold the eyelids open and flood the eye with water for 15 minutes.

(c) After flooding the eye with water, ask someone in the household to contact the police, fire, or emergency squad.

(d) Cover the eye with a sterile pad—***do not use cotton***—to keep the lid from moving.

(e) Notify Home Care Supervisor.

17. Identify actions to be taken in case of bleeding injury.
    a. If the cut is small, follow these steps.
        1) Inform the parent(s). Show the wound but do not touch the wound until your hands have been washed.
        2) Wash your hands.
        3) Wash the wound thoroughly with soap and water.
        4) Cover the wound with a bandage, being careful not to touch the gauze area with your fingers.
    b. If the wound is bleeding heavily and/or the injury is extensive, take the following measures.
        1) Have the victim lie down.
        2) Inform the household and have someone contact the police, fire, or emergency squad.
        3) Control the bleeding by applying pressure to pressure points. (Note illustrations.)

18. Identify the actions to be taken with a postpartum mother who is experiencing excessive bleeding/hemorrhage.
    a. Assist the mother to bed.
    b. Assist the mother to locate and massage the fundus of uterus.
    c. Request the physician's number and contact immediately for instructions.
    d. Call the police, fire, or emergency squad if instructed to do so by the physician.
    e. Inquire if you should call a family member.
    f. Notify Home Care Supervisor.

19. Identify the procedure to be followed if a mother requests your advice concerning a suspected physical problem.
    a. Show concern; ask the mother if she would like to sit or lie down.
    b. Depending on the mother's condition, request that she discuss the problem with the physician/practitioner. If the woman's condition warrants, call the physician for her.
    c. Assist the mother to follow the physician/practitioner's instructions.
    d. Notify Home Care Supervisor.

20. List 12 effective safety measures in the kitchen.
    a. Never leave cooking items unattended; this may cause a fire. If you are distracted, turn off the gas or electric burner before leaving the room.
    b. Always keep pot handles turned in toward the stove. Young children may reach up and pull hot food onto themselves.

c. Always keep the electric cords of cooking equipment (electric frying pans, coffeepots, etc.) out of children's reach.

d. Always keep hot liquids out of a baby's reach. Children in this age group are the most frequent victims of hot liquid scalds. In a split second they can grab a coffee cup or bump your arm.

e. Keep tablecloth ends up on the table. Toddlers can spill hot liquids by pulling at the edges of a tablecloth.

f. Protect babies or toddlers by placing them in a high chair or playpen during cooking hours.

g. If a grease, fat, lard, or cooking oil fire starts, ***do not use water*** to extinguish it. Smother the fire by covering it with a lid or use a dry chemical-type fire extinguisher if available. (Baking soda will also work.)

h. Take care that curtains near kitchen ranges and heating equipment do not catch fire.

i. Store cookies, cereals, or other children's "bait" away from the stove because children may be burned reaching for them.

j. Extinguish oven fires by closing the oven door and turning off the heat or by using a dry chemical-type fire extinguisher. (Baking soda will also work.)

k. Do not use a gas range to heat the room, for the following reasons.

   1) You may initiate a fire.

   2) The oxygen in the air may be used up.

l. Never place any type of metal in a microwave oven, including foil, metal pots and pans, and dishes with silver or gold trim. Check the safety of cooking utensils with the parent(s).

21. List other safety measures for preventing accidental burn injury.

   a. Home Health Aides are not permitted to smoke in clients' homes. Make sure ashtrays used by clients or guests are wet thoroughly with water before emptying and cleaning.

   b. Keep matches away from heat sources such as ranges or heaters.

   c. Do not use multiple electrical attachment plugs, and avoid use of long extension cords.

   d. Do not run extension cords under rugs, through doorways or partitions, or over hooks, radiators, heaters, pipes, or ducts.

   e. If the family is using space heaters, select a safe location away from traffic, children, and flammable materials.

MODULE 2: HOUSEHOLD MANAGEMENT

Describe specific activities necessary for effective household management and organizational skills required to accomplish expected tasks.

1. Identify specific activities to assist client in Self-Care Approach. (See Box 3-1.)
   a. Introduce suggested Self-Care Approach guidelines to client during interview.
   b. Inform client to make you aware of any items you could carry out to assist her.
   c. Explain to client that the Self-Care Approach guidelines are only a suggested tool to assist her in organizing her needs.
   d. Identify housekeeping tasks that will be expected of you. (These tasks will vary from home to home.)
      1) Preparing meals
      2) Washing, folding, and/or putting away laundry
      3) Wiping up spilled food
      4) Sweeping, vacuuming, and mopping floors
      5) Dusting
      6) Cleaning bathroom sink, tub, and/or toilet
      7) Taking out garbage
      8) Wiping kitchen countertops, tables, and sinks
      9) Wiping top of range
      10) Checking refrigerator and freezer for spoiled food
      11) Washing dishes
      12) Changing bed linens
      13) Reporting safety hazards to client
2. Identify objectives relating to effective and organized meal preparation.
   a. Identify meals to be prepared and served.
   b. Locate food items, plan menu for day, and plan preparation of food.
   c. Check ingredients on food packages to be sure no one in the house will have an allergic reaction. (The client should inform you of any allergies beforehand.)
   d. Identify and organize all equipment needed for cooking.
   e. Review instructions before use of any electrical equipment.
   f. Determine proper use of range/oven.
   g. Determine time required to cook each item, and schedule cooking times so the entire meal is finished at once.
   h. Organize food items necessary for meal.
   i. Begin meal preparation.
   j. While meal is cooking, set necessary trays and table for family.
   k. Serve warm meal to family. Do not place hot foods in front of young children.
   l. Practice safety knowledge acquired in Module 1.

BOX 3-1: FAMILY HELP, INC.—CLIENT SELF-CARE APPROACH GUIDELINES

The self-care approach is health oriented. Emphasis is concentrated on the needs of the "whole" client and recognizes your ability to be an active decision-maker in the process of returning to the regular activities of daily living. It is based on the idea of looking into yourself and reflecting on your environment and experiences. The following are only suggested guidelines that may assist you in adapting to the new demands and changes that occur during this time. Please advise us if we may be of assistance in helping you develop or carry out your plan.

Write a list—

1. Express your feelings, listing them all. (You may be feeling happy, comfortable, exhausted, angry, sad, overwhelmed, out of control, and so on.)
2. Next to each feeling on your list, describe what you think may be some of the reasons causing you to have these feelings.

   EXAMPLES:

   - Happy—Think about the things you are doing that give you the most happiness.
   - Sad—Identify those feeling that cause the most worry, guilt, or concern (e.g., "I'm not spending enough time with my children . . . ," "My house is a wreck . . . , " "I miss my job . . . ")
   - Comfortable—Identify those things that make you feel rested, peaceful, content, etc.
   - Exhausted—How much rest and sleep are you actually getting, and what are you doing while awake?
   - Overwhelmed—List it all! Everyone and everything that is drawing on your energy (e.g., "This baby is so demanding—I just can't do it. . . . ")
   - Out of control—List all the things that upset you that you feel you can't do anything about.
   - Inadequate—Have you set yourself unreasonably high standards as to what kind of mother you think you "should" be?
3. Express your needs and identify exactly what you feel to be *your* needs if you are to regain your physical strength and make family adjustments.
4. List things to do based on your feelings and needs.
   a. Items that promote rest and "good feelings" should be listed under "things to do."
   b. Items that cause distress should be listed under "things to get help for."
5. Identify possible sources of assistance (e.g., family, friends, physician/practitioner, nanny, homemaker).
6. Verbalize your needs and plan with family member, friend, nurse, or homemaker if you feel the need to do so.
7. Enlist all sources of help, and identify clearly for these people exactly what it is they can do for you (e.g., watch infant and/or other children while you rest; bring a meal). If the people around you are unsure of what it is that you want or need, they may not be as helpful as they could potentially be.
8. List tasks for which you can't get help.
   a. Identify the importance of each task and decide if it is essential that it be done.
   b. Determine how you can get these tasks done to create more ease for you (e.g., setting up baby-changing stations throughout the house, preplanning meals, developing a schedule that allows you to rest when the children are resting).

3. Identify six elements in the proper use of cleaning agents.
   a. Always read labels carefully to see which products may be used for a particular surface or item.
   b. Use each product only as stated on the label.
   c. If mixing with water is necessary, mix according to directions.
   d. Never mix cleaning products together—this may produce dangerous fumes.
   e. Never use bleach in household cleaning.
   f. Practice safety knowledge acquired in Module 1.

4. Explain nine elements necessary for proper laundering of clothes.
   a. Always check clothing labels to determine if machine washable and machine dryable.
   b. Sort clothing according to color, fabric, and washing instructions.
   c. Hot wash–cold rinse: Use for regular whites and *colorfast* (nonfading) loads, especially if heavily soiled and/or with greasy or oily stains. Diapers are always rinsed of any stool or urine first and washed separately from other clothes. Rinse twice.
   d. Warm wash–cold rinse: Use for permanent press and special care fabrics (polyester, nylon, or acrylic). Also, use to help preserve bright or dark colors. Hand wash delicate items in warm water.
   e. Cold wash–cold rinse: Use for dark or bright colors that fade and for some stains, such as blood or chocolate. Hot water causes stains to set in the fabric, so *use cold water* to keep tough stains like these from staining clothes permanently.
   f. Use the right amount of detergent.
      1) Top-loading automatics
         (a) Normal capacity: 1 cup
         (b) Large capacity: $1\frac{1}{3}$ to $1\frac{1}{2}$ cups
      2) Front-loading automatics: Start with $\frac{1}{3}$ to $\frac{1}{2}$ cup or enough to bring suds $\frac{1}{3}$ to $\frac{1}{2}$ up the window.
      3) Portable washers: $\frac{1}{3}$ to $\frac{1}{2}$ cup
   g. Add detergent to dispenser or put in the machine before the clothing.
   h. Dry according to instructions on clothing labels.
   i. Always follow any specific instructions of client.

MODULE 3: INFECTION CONTROL

This section covers actions the Family-Centered Home Health Aide can undertake to assist in preventing the spread of infection. Upon completion of this unit, the learner should be prepared to accomplish the following.

1. Explain the term "infection."
   The state or condition in which the body, or a part of it, is invaded by a pathogenic agent (disease-producing microorganism or virus), which, under conditions favorable to the agent, multiplies and produces effects that are injurious (germ-caused illness).

2. Explain the term "organism."
   Any living thing—plant or animal. Organisms may be one-celled (bacteria, yeasts, protozoans) "germs" or many-celled individuals (such as humans).

3. Explain the term "normal flora."
   Resident organisms (germs) in a particular area that do not usually cause disease in the host. (We carry many germs that may not cause us to become ill, yet when spread to someone else may cause illness in him or her.)

4. Explain the term "host."
   A host is a living organism from which another organism receives its nourishment. (Our bodies are host to many organisms, which for the most part do not make us ill—they are our "normal flora.")

5. Explain the term "source of infection."
   The human, animal, or environmental home for the organism (germ) from which human infection is usually derived. (A person who sneezes into his hand then shakes someone else's hand may be that second person's source of infection.)

6. Explain the term "spread of infection."
   The way in which organisms (germs) are transferred from a source to a susceptible human host.

7. Define the word "susceptible" as it applies here.
   "Susceptible," in this instance, means having a lowered ability to fight off infection.

8. Identify factors that may affect and lower our ability to fight off infection.
   a. Age and sex (Babies and the elderly have less ability to fight off infection.)
   b. Improper nutrition
   c. Presence of disease
   d. Blood loss
   e. Certain medications
   f. Fatigue
   g. Generally poor physical condition

9. Identify the common practices that help prevent the spread of organisms (germs), thus preventing the possible spread of infection.
   a. Washing hands is the most important way to prevent the spread of organisms (germs).

b. Keep soiled items and/or equipment from touching clothing; carry soiled linens so they do not touch your uniform.

c. Clean away from yourself and the family, especially when brushing, dusting, or scrubbing articles. This prevents particles from settling on your (or others') hair, face, or uniform.

d. Clean least soiled areas first, and then the more soiled ones.

e. Avoid raising dust, because dust particles may transport organisms (germs).

10. Explain proper handwashing technique and practice.

    a. When arriving on the job, all Home Health Aides should wash their hands thoroughly for 2 minutes up to the elbows. Soap, warm water, and friction when rubbing hands together are the key to removing most organisms that are on the skin. Hands are the most common way in which germs are spread. When washing, use the warmest water you can tolerate, taking care not to burn yourself. Start at the elbows and work your way down to the hands.

    b. When rinsing, direct hands downward into the sink to rinse off soap, starting from the elbows. Remember, most germs need to be scrubbed off because they can attach themselves to the skin. Repeat this procedure for 1 minute before and after meals, after working with laundry, after touching your nose, mouth, hair, or after using the telephone. (Please note: No personal calls.)

    c. Always wash your hands before caring for the mother or her baby, before serving meals to the family, and after using the bathroom (wash for 2 minutes). Wash your hands before leaving your job to go home.

11. Identify infection control principles for routine handling of soiled linens in the home.

    a. It is not routinely necessary if good handwashing is observed, but it is recommended that you obtain gloves and use them when handling dirty linens. Always wash hands using the proper technique after handling laundry.

    b. Carry soiled laundry away from your body so as not to touch your uniform. Use a laundry basket if one is available.

    c. Soiled laundry should be handled as little as possible to prevent germs from being carried into the air and to protect the person handling the laundry.

12. State the requirements of the dress code.

    a. Carry your clean uniform to the job in some type of carryall bag.

    b. Explain to the client the need to change into your uniform on the job so that no "street germs" are brought into contact with either the family or the newborn.

    c. Wear proper undergarments.

    d. Limit jewelry to small, "dot," post earrings and wedding rings only. No jewelry is preferable, because rings can carry germs.

    e. Hair should be pulled back if it is mid-neck length or longer.

    f. Wear plain, solid-colored knee socks or white or beige stockings only.

    g. Wear closed-toed shoes—no clogs, thongs, or sandals.

MODULE 4: COMMUNICATION

This section covers aspects of effective communication between the Family-Centered Home Health Aide and the client. Upon completion of this unit, the learner should be prepared to accomplish the following.

1. Discuss initial protocols for establishing a relationship with your client.
   a. Identify yourself by name.
   b. Specify your reason for being there.
   c. Identify by name the agency sending you and your job title.
   d. Indicate your need to spend some time with the client and/or family to discuss the plan of care.
   e. State specifically how much time you need to spend. Request 15 minutes for you and the client and/or family members to sit and develop their plan of care.
   f. Discuss the individual client's special needs and document them on the Home Health Aide's plan of care.
   g. Review Client Rights: Terms and Conditions and clarify for the client.
   h. Request that the client review the developed plan and sign the indicated area if in agreement.
   i. Use positive communication techniques.
   j. Give client educational pamphlets and Guidelines for Self-Care Approach.
   k. Initiate the Helping Relationship. (See Box 3-2.)
2. Identify positive and negative communication techniques and give examples of each.
   a. Positive communication techniques
      1) Using silence permits the client to talk about what he or she wishes.
      2) Accepting: "Yes." "Um humm." "I follow what you said." Nodding.
      3) Giving recognition: "Good morning, Mr. B." "You've tooled a leather wallet." "I notice you've done your hair."

BOX 3-2: THE HELPING RELATIONSHIP

Orientation Phase: The client will know the nurse by name and accurately describe the roles of the participants in the relationship. The client and nurse will establish an agreement regarding:

- Goals of the relationship
- Location, frequency, and length of contact

Working Phase: The nurse and client work together to meet the client's goals. The client actively participates, cooperating in activities to reach those goals. The client can express his or her feelings and concerns to the nurse.

Termination: The client participates in identifying progress toward or accomplishment of goals. The client verbalizes feelings about the termination of the relationship.

4) Offering self: "I'll sit with you awhile." "I'll stay here with you." "I'm interested in your comfort."

5) Giving broad openings: "Is there something you'd like to talk about?" "What are you thinking about?" "Where would you like to begin?"

6) Placing the event in time or in sequence: "What seemed to lead up to . . . ?" "Was this before or after . . . ?" "When did this happen?"

7) Making observations: "You appear tense." "Are you uncomfortable when you . . . ?" "I notice that you're biting your lips."

8) Restating: Client: "I can't sleep. I stay awake all night." Caregiver: "You have difficulty sleeping?"

9) Reflecting: Client: "No, you think I should tell the doctor?" Caregiver: "Do you think you should?"

   Or: Client: "My brother spends all my money and then has the nerve to ask for more." Caregiver: "This makes you feel angry."

10) Focusing: "This point seems worth looking at more closely."

11) Exploring: "Tell me more about that. . . . " "Would you describe it more fully?" "What kind of work?"

12) Giving information: "My name is. . . . My purpose in being here is. . . . I'm taking you to the. . . . "

13) Seeking clarification: "I'm not sure that I follow. . . . " "What would you say is the main point of what you said?"

14) Giving support: "You are so organized." "You are really making progress."

15) Open-ended statements give the client an opening to continue verbalizing: Client: "First, I felt dizzy." Caregiver: "And then?" or "And after that?"

b. Negative communication techniques

1) Giving approval (avoid making value judgments): "That's good. I'm glad that you. . . . "

2) Rejecting: "Let's not discuss. . . . " "I don't want to hear about. . . . "

3) Disapproving: "That's bad." "I'd rather you wouldn't."

4) Agreeing: "That's right." "I agree."

5) Disagreeing: "That's wrong." "I definitely disagree with. . . . " "I don't believe that."

6) Advising: "I think you should. . . . " "Why don't you . . . ?"

7) Making stereotyped comments: "Nice weather we're having." "I'm fine. And how are you?" "It's for your own good." "Keep your chin up." "Just listen to your doctor and take part in activities." "You'll be better in no time."

8) Using denial: Client: "I'm nothing." Caregiver: "Of course you're something."

   Or: Client: "I can't do it." Caregiver: "Don't be silly."

9) Interpreting: "What you really mean is. . . . " "Unconsciously you're saying. . . . "

10) Introducing an unrelated topic: Client: "I'd like to cry." Caregiver: "Did you have visitors this weekend?"

MODULE 5: NEWBORN CARE

This section covers actions the Family-Centered Home Health Aide can undertake to promote safe and healthy care of the newborn. Upon completion of this unit, the learner should be prepared to accomplish the following.

1. Identify the goal of family-centered care during the postpartum period.
   The goal of family-centered care is to maintain and support the needs and desires of each individual family. "Family" may represent the traditional mother/father/child unit or may represent those persons participating in family roles of providing love, support, and care of mother, infant, and other children.

2. Identify the physical needs and endowments of the newborn.
   a. Sensation
      1) The infant's first impressions of life are derived mainly through the sense of touch.
      2) Touch should convey to the infant feelings of security, pleasure, and love.
      3) Touching the infant in certain locations will cause reflex responses, depending on the area touched (e.g., stroking the cheek elicits rooting reflex, touching the mouth triggers the sucking reflex, touching the palm or hand activates the grasp reflex).

   b. Vision
      1) The infant is aware of differences in light. His or her eyes may follow large moving objects.
      2) The infant has difficulty focusing his or her eyes.

   c. Hearing
      1) The infant will respond to conversation-level sound.
      2) Loud noises will evoke a startle response.

   d. Taste: Sense of taste and smell are not well developed.

   e. Motor activity
      1) Head control is poorly developed, although the head may be turned from side to side. The head needs support from the caregiver's hand until the infant reaches 4 months of age.
      2) The extremities (arms and legs) are drawn up close to the body.
      3) The infant may exhibit many movements and should never be left alone on a couch, bed, or similar surface from which he or she may fall.

3. Identify the infant's needs for stimulation of the senses in relationship to proper growth and development.
   a. Studies indicate that infant nerve pathways are immature and must be stimulated to function adequately.
   b. Adequate stimulation is provided through the following means.
      1) Soothing
      2) Holding
      3) Flocking

4) Changing position
5) Stroking the skin
6) Singing, playing music, and talking
7) Visual stimulation can be achieved by changing patterns of light and shade.

4. Describe how infants demonstrate individual differences from birth.
   a. Activity level: Some infants are very active from the time of birth, whereas others may be, for the most part, passive or quiet.
   b. Sensitivity: Infants may demonstrate individual preferences for stimulation of their senses: for example, some may respond consistently to touching whereas others may be more responsive to singing.
   c. Self-stimulation: Some infants may engage in constant mouth activity (e.g., sucking, hands in mouth).
   d. Patterns of sleep/waking/feeding: Some babies develop regular patterns, and others may be more unpredictable.

5. Identify situations that may cause the infant to signal discomfort/distress. These situations need investigation. Crying is the infant's signal for help. The following are sources of distress to be checked if the infant cries.
   a. Hunger
      1) Determine time since the last feeding. Newborns feed usually every 3 to 4 hours, some even 2 to 3 hours. Do not wake a sleeping infant.
      2) Check rooting and sucking reflexes with clean fingers. Hungry infants will quickly respond.
   b. Soiled diapers
      If diaper is wet or soiled, gather equipment necessary for diaper change. Have the baby in a protected area such as the crib, cradle, or an adult's arms.
      1) Wash your hands.
      2) Use a warm washcloth or premoistened baby wipes, whichever the parent(s) prefer.
      3) You will need a diaper.
      4) Ask the parent(s) if they use ointment (e.g., A&D ointment), always checking the label for proper use before applying to the baby.
      5) If cloth diapers are used, only use diaper pins with safety heads.
      6) If disposable diapers are used, the side with the sticky tabs is placed under the baby's back.
      7) Lay the baby on a flat surface.
      8) Keep your hand on the baby at all times.
      9) Remove the soiled diaper.
      10) Wipe away soil with a cloth.
      11) Clean the baby's skin gently but thoroughly.
      12) Pay special attention to skin folds and creases when cleaning, drying, and applying ointments.
      13) Wipe soil away from the genital area toward the anal region (front to back).

14) Put on the clean diaper and fold the diaper so as not to cover the umbilical area.
15) Provide care for umbilicus (navel) as indicated by client.
16) Provide safe place for infant.
17) Clean up the diaper-changing area.
18) Rinse soiled diapers in toilet. Cloth diapers should be placed in the diaper pail or disposed of in waste. ***Never flush in toilet.***

c. Uncomfortable body position: Try holding the baby in different positions.
   1) Upright position: Hold the baby with your left forearm supporting the him or her under the buttocks. Press his or her body against your shoulder and chest. The infant's cheek should rest against your left shoulder. Use your right hand to support the head and neck.
   2) Football hold: Support the baby's head in the palm of your left hand. The baby's back is supported along your left forearm. His or her hips will be pressed against your waist by your left elbow, holding the baby securely in place. You may use either arm for this hold as long as you support the head and back.
   3) Cradle position: Slide your left hand and arm under the baby's back and use your left arm to support head, back, and bottom. With your right hand under the baby's buttocks, move your left arm and hand toward the baby's head while picking him or her up. Cradle the baby, holding him or her against your chest, the left arm supporting the head, back, and shoulders, and the right arm supporting the buttocks, legs, and feet.

d. Fatigue: Lay the baby in a crib or cradle on back or side with head turned to side. Other relief measures to try follow.
   1) Hold the baby securely and rock to sleep.
   2) Pat or rub the baby's back with a steady rhythm.
   3) Provide a quiet area for sleep.

e. Extremes of temperature
   1) Check the temperature of the home.
   2) Check to be sure that the baby is not in a draft.
   3) Determine if the baby is too hot or too cold by feeling the baby's skin.
   4) If the baby is too hot, try the following measures.
      (a) Sponge with a cool (not cold) washcloth.
      (b) Change clothing if excessive or if damp; try to locate cool, summery, cotton clothing.
      (c) If the baby is hot for environmental reasons, consult with the parent(s). The infant's temperature should be taken to determine if illness is possible cause.
   5) If the baby is too cold, wrap snugly in a blanket, removing him from any household drafts.

f. Abdominal distension
   1) Attempt to determine the reason for the distension. (See Module 1, Safety-Promoting Activities, objective 13.)
   2) If there are no signs or symptoms of emergency, look for other possible reasons.

(a) The infant may be experiencing gas pains. Try burping by holding the baby in effective positions for burping. Pat or stroke the infant's back while keeping his or her stomach close to part of your body.

- Try the upright hold described above.
- A sitting position may be helpful. Place the baby on your lap facing sideways, allowing one hand to soothe and support the baby's abdomen. Use the thumb and index area of the same hand to support the baby's head under the chin. Gently but firmly pat or rub baby's back with the other hand.
- Another effective position is over the knees. Place the baby over the knees, keeping the head up on the knees. Gently but firmly pat or stroke the baby's back. Hold the baby's body firmly with the other hand.

(b) Attempt to soothe the baby by walking, rocking, holding securely, and/or stroking the skin.

(c) The infant may just want to be held and cuddled. This is a very important need that all infants have. Gently hold and cuddle the infant.

6. Define the purpose, composition, care, and possible complications of the umbilical cord.
   a. The umbilical cord functions as the lifeline, connecting the fetus with the mother's placenta, allowing for the exchange of oxygen and nutrients.
   b. It is composed of a jelly-like substance that begins to dry when exposed to the air. At delivery, it is clamped and cut. Within 7 to 10 days the stump will dry, turn black, and fall off.
   c. The client(s) will have been given specific instructions in cord care by the physician/practitioner/nurse. Most instructions include the use of a drying agent such as alcohol with each diaper change. Verify client's protocol at the initial interview before applying anything to the infant's skin. Document on Homemaker's Plan of Care. If a drying agent is used, dab on the cord gently, covering the entire area.
   d. ***Never*** pull on the cord. Let it fall off by itself. Laying the infant on the abdomen will not hurt the cord. Use of binders or belly bands is not recommended.
   e. Problems with the cord that should be reported to the client, who should consult with physician/practitioner, include the following.
      1) Foul odor of cord area
      2) Purulent material (pus)
      3) Bleeding, other than a few drops when the cord falls off
      4) Red and sore appearance; skin around area warmer than usual
   f. Do not allow the diaper to cover the cord area because this will delay the drying process. If allowed to be wet, the cord may become infected.

7. Describe the principles and procedures for an infant sponge bath.
   a. The infant may not receive a tub bath until the cord has fallen off.
   b. Obtain items needed for a bath.
      1) Use mild soap to prevent skin irritation. Consult with the client on this and document on the Homemaker's Plan of Care.
      2) You will need two or three towels or receiving blankets for drying the infant.
      3) Have two washcloths handy.

4) Use two basins or two large bowls or pots as available in the home.
5) Be sure to get the baby's clothes ready before the bath: diaper, undershirt, clothes/sleeper, blanket.
6) You will need ointment as indicated by the client for circumcision care.
7) You will need cord care items as indicated by the client.
8) Spread the towel(s) on a safe table or carpeted floor space out of any air draft. This will provide a clean, warm spot for the baby and prevent the carpet or bed from becoming wet.

c. Sponging procedures
   1) Fill basins with warm water (***never hot***; test with your elbow).
   2) Use one basin for soapy water and for rinsing the soapy washcloth.
   3) Use one basin for clear water and the soapless washcloth.
   4) Only one part of the infant's body is washed at a time, taking care to keep other parts of the body covered to prevent chill.
   5) Use only clear, soapless water and washcloth on the baby's face. Eyes are wiped from inside corner outward. Use a different corner of the cloth for each eye.
   6) Wash the infant's head using gentle circular motions to prevent cradle cap from forming.
   7) Wash the rest of the infant's body one area at a time with mild soap and water; rinse with clear water and cloth from soapless basin. Talking and smiling reassuringly to the baby throughout the bath will make it a pleasant experience.
   8) Dry the infant well as each part of body is finished being rinsed.
      (a) Special areas to check include: behind ears, under and around the neck, creases around the eyes, underside of the arm at the shoulder, backsides of the knees, ankle creases, in between toes and fingers, creases inside the thighs and under buttocks. Around the genital area, separate the infant girl's labia and pat dry, front to back; for boys, dry the underside of the scrotum.
      (b) Improper drying can cause irritation and chafing of skin, which could contribute to skin infections in the infant.
      (c) Always keep one hand on the baby throughout the bathing process.
   9) Dress the baby and lay in a safe, warm place on the stomach or side. Always direct the baby's head to the side.
   10) Clean up the equipment and return everything to its proper place.

8. Describe the principles and procedures for an infant tub bath. This procedure must also be used when bathing older babies.
   a. Obtain the necessary items.
      1) Determine the place of the bath (e.g., infant tub, sink, bathtub).
      2) Use mild soap to prevent skin irritation. Identify with the client initially and document on Homemaker's Plan of Care.
      3) Obtain two towels, one large enough to completely wrap the baby.
      4) You will need one washcloth.
      5) Be sure you have ointment as specified by the client for circumcision care.

b. Wash the area where the baby will be bathed (tub, sink, etc.). If using the tub or sink, place a small towel in the bottom to prevent the baby from slipping.

c. Take the phone off the hook and replace after the bath unless the mother is awake and willing to accept phone calls.

d. Fill the bath with warm water, testing with your elbow, and review the safety objectives in Module 1 for bathing the baby.

e. Hold the infant in the cradle position and immerse in the warm bath.

f. Wash each part of the infant's body and rinse with plenty of water. ***Never turn the faucets on while the infant is in the bath.*** Do not use soap on the face.

g. Wash the infant's head, using a gentle circular motion to help prevent cradle cap. Hold the head back so that soap and rinsing water will not get into the eyes.

h. Wrap the infant in a towel and dry very carefully, paying special attention to the areas in objective 7 above, sections a through c.

i. Dress the infant and lay him or her in a safe place on the abdomen or side with the head turned to the side. Keep warm.

j. Straighten up the bath area, wring out any wet towels thoroughly, and dry as appropriate.

9. Explain the procedures and rationale for the care of circumcision.

   a. Determine from the client when the circumcision was performed.

   b. When changing the diaper, report to the client any blood stains in the diaper or any foul odor so that the physician/practitioner may be informed per instructions.

   c. Apply ointment or Vaseline liberally as the client has been instructed by the physician/practitioner. Document the instructions on the Home Health Aide's Plan of Care. Most instructions suggest using a large dab of A&D ointment or Vaseline on the circumcised area of the penis to prevent this sore area from sticking to the diaper and to promote healing.

10. Explain the types of infant formula, their preparation, and proper use.
    Identify the type of formula and instructions for preparation. Consult with the client regarding the usual amount of formula the infant takes at a meal. Document the information on the Homemaker's Plan of Care. Note the expiration date on the can, and do not use if the date has passed.

    a. Ready to feed: No mixing with water is required.

    b. Concentrated liquid: Requires mixing with equal parts of water (e.g., one ounce of water mixed with one ounce of formula).

    c. Powdered mix: Requires mixing with water. Follow the instructions on the package.

    d. Soy protein formulas: Prepare according to the package instructions; indicated for babies sensitive to cow's milk. These are available in ready to feed, concentrated, or powdered forms.

    e. Ounce measurements should be made accurately. If a calibrated pitcher is unavailable, use a clean bottle to measure the proper number of ounces of water and formula.

11. Discuss with the client the physician/practitioner's instructions concerning the need for sterilization of bottles and water.

    a. Wash your hands well.

    b. If sterilization of bottles is not required, clean the bottles and nipples vigorously with soap and water, rinsing thoroughly.

c. If sterilization of water is not necessary, mix tap water with formula as indicated and according to instructions.

d. If preparing bottles of formula for storage, always use boiled water for mixing to decrease the growth of bacteria (germs).

e. If sterilization of equipment is necessary, follow this procedure.

    1) Identify the type of equipment to be used. If a commercial sterilizer, review the instructions for its proper use. If sterilizing of equipment is to be done on the stove, assemble the following equipment and then continue with the sterilization procedure.

        (a) Nipples
        (b) Bottle brush
        (c) Dishwashing detergent
        (d) Hot water from tap
        (e) Large pot with cover
        (f) Small towel
        (g) Tap water
        (h) Timer, watch, or clock
        (i) Tongs
        (j) Clean, empty jar

    2) Wash your hands.

    3) Scrub the bottles, nipples, and caps with hot soapy water. Squirt water through the nipple holes to clean out any dried formula.

    4) Rinse well with hot water.

    5) Fold a small towel to fit the bottom of the pot and lay it there to prevent the bottles from breaking. (Use a towel only if there is no bottle rack available.)

    6) Place caps and nipples into a clean empty jar. Place it into the pot at the center of the bottles.

    7) Pour water into and around the bottles and into the jar holding the nipples and caps until each bottle is $^{2}/_{3}$ filled.

    8) Cover the pot.

    9) Place the pot on the burner and turn burner setting to high or full.

    10) Begin timing for 25 minutes after the water comes to a full boil. Remove the nipples and caps after 15 minutes.

    11) After 25 minutes, turn off the burner.

    12) Take the cover off the pot and allow it to cool.

    13) Remove the bottles with tongs. Do not touch the tops or insides of the bottles.

    14) Prepare the formula, place formula in bottles, place nipples and caps on bottles tightly, and cover. Store in the refrigerator.

f. Never use formula stored in the refrigerator for longer than 2 days.

g. Formula that has been unrefrigerated for longer than 1 hour begins to spoil. Dispose of any formula left out for more than an hour and begin with a fresh preparation.

h. Remove the chill from the bottle by placing in a pot of hot tap water for several minutes. Do not heat on the stove.

i. Always test the temperature of the formula on your wrist before feeding to avoid scalding the infant's mouth.

j. Explain the procedure for sterilizing tap water.

1) Assemble the following equipment.

(a) Saucepan

(b) Water

(c) Timer, watch, or clock

2) Wash your hands.

3) Fill the saucepan until it is 2/3 full of water.

4) Place the covered saucepan on the stove and turn the burner to the high setting.

5) Once the water comes to full boil, set the timer for 20 minutes.

6) Turn off the burner and allow the water to cool before mixing.

12. Identify the purpose, equipment, and procedure for infant bottle feeding.

a. Purpose

1) To supply proper nourishment to the baby.

2) To provide fluid intake in adequate amounts.

b. Equipment

1) Formula at room temperature

2) Two diapers and ointment as instructed by client

c. Procedure (Bottle-fed infants usually demand feedings every 3 to 4 hours.)

1) Wash hands and dry thoroughly.

2) Change the diaper.

3) Wrap the infant in a receiving blanket and put a bib on him or her (a clean diaper can be used as a bib).

4) Wash your hands after changing the diaper.

5) Position the baby in a sitting position for feeding.

(a) Hold the bottle at such an angle that the nipple is always full to avoid the swallowing of air.

(b) Burp the baby after taking 1/2 to 1 ounce.

6) Position the baby for burping, using one of following techniques.

(a) Keeping baby in an upright position, place the baby's chin in the palm of your hand and gently pat the baby on the back with your other hand.

(b) Place a clean diaper on your shoulder and hold the baby in an upright position with the head resting on your shoulder securely and gently pat the baby on the back until he or she burps.

7) Change the diaper and crib sheet if necessary.

8) Place the baby on his or her abdomen in the crib unless otherwise instructed.

9) Chart the date, time, intake, stools, and urine on the Homemaker's Progress Note.
10) Rinse and discard the bottles; clean up the work areas.
11) Wash and dry your hands thoroughly.
12) Report any feeding difficulties to the client and document on the Homemaker's Progress Note.

13. Discuss the importance of breastfeeding.
    a. Mother's milk is the best food for the normal newborn.
    b. Nutritional, health, and emotional benefits exist for both the mother and the baby.
    c. Breast milk supplies the full range of nutrients to satisfy baby's growth and development needs.
    d. Infants digest mother's milk easily.
    e. Breast milk offers the baby protection against some infections. Colostrum, the yellowish or white fluid that is the "first milk" contains antibodies that protect the infant against certain infections.
    f. Breastfeeding promotes the bonding of mother and child through the intimate relationship that develops.

14. Discuss common breastfeeding techniques and points to remember when the mother requests assistance with feeding.
    a. Wash your hands.
    b. Assist the mother to assume a comfortable position.
    c. Encourage the mother to help the baby start nursing by holding him or her close so that the baby's cheek touches the breast.
    d. The baby should take as much of the areola (the darker area surrounding the nipple) as possible into his or her mouth, not just the nipple. The nipple should be erect; the mother may need to roll an inverted nipple between her thumb and index finger to make it protrude.
    e. If the mother's breast is full, explain to her that using one finger to press the breast away from the infant's nose will allow easier breathing for the baby.
    f. Encourage the mother to use both breasts and to alternate the side she begins with; a safety pin fastened to the bra strap may help to remind her.
    g. Never pull the nipple from the baby's mouth. To break suction, press the breast away from the corner of the mouth or lift the baby's lip by putting a clean finger into the corner of the mouth.
    h. The baby should be burped after feedings.
    i. A nursing bra may provide comfortable support.
    j. Encourage the mother to leave the nursing flaps of her bra down whenever possible to allow the nipples to dry. Allow the nipples to dry before applying any cream recommended by the physician/practitioner.
    k. The mother may ask questions about cramping during nursing. This is nature's way of returning the uterus to its normal size.
    l. Breastfed babies may desire nursing every 2 to 3 hours.
    m. The mother's milk supply will increase with an increased amount of nursing.

n. Do not use soap or antiseptics on the nipples as they tend to cause excessive drying of the skin.

o. Encourage the mother to drink 10 glasses of water daily to help keep her supply of milk adequate, and to avoid caffeine and tobacco. Caffeine and nicotine eventually enter the mother's milk and are consumed by the baby.

p. Six or more wet diapers a day assures the mother that her baby is getting enough milk.

q. Support and encourage mothers in breastfeeding. "We must identify and reduce barriers which keep women from beginning or continuing to breastfeed their infants." C. Everett Koop, M.D., Sc.D., former Surgeon General.

15. Identify positions that may assist the mother to relax while breastfeeding.

    a. Lying on her side with a pillow under her head, one arm may be positioned above her head while the other arm may be used to cradle the baby.

    b. If sitting, use a chair with a back support. The baby's head and back can be supported in the bend of her elbow.

16. Identify variations of the normal newborn that the Home Health Aide may note.

    a. Skin

        1) The normal skin color at birth skin may be purplish red. Within the next few days, skin becomes the typical pink. Mottling (red streaking) may appear if the infant is cold. A pink color at rest may become red when the baby cries. Flaking of the skin may occur.

        2) Jaundice in the newborn

            (a) One-third to one-half of all newborns develop jaundice in the first week.

            (b) Causes: Increased destruction of red blood cells no longer needed after birth and immaturity of the liver.

            (c) Jaundice is most readily seen on the face and brow. It may also be seen in the whites of the eyes.

            (d) Press your finger down on the skin of the cheek, brow, and chest. Note the color of the skin as you lift finger immediately. This may allow the yellow hue to become more visible.

            (e) If a yellow color is noted, notify the client that the physician/practitioner should be made aware of the condition.

            (f) Ill effects are rare, but jaundice may cause sleepiness and lack of interest in feeding.

        3) Milia are tiny oil cysts, appearing as white, pinhead-sized spots, mainly on and around the nose.

        4) Forceps marks are bruised areas on the face. These will disappear within a few days, and problems are rare.

        5) Newborn rash may occur, where small areas (1 to 2 cm) of redness may appear, resembling flea bites. The center may contain a small, raised, yellowish spot. The infant is not ill and treatment is rarely necessary.

    b. Head

        1) Moulding is the way in which the bones of the head have changed during birth to allow the baby to fit through the passageway. The baby may have a "conehead" appearance. The head will return to its normal shape within a few days.

2) The client should be aware of any problems of the head and face and instructed in care by the physician/practitioner. It is your responsibility to follow the instructions given by the client. If in doubt, consult the Home Care Supervisor.

c. Eyes

1) An infant's eyes may normally appear "cross-eyed."

2) Hemorrhages (blood spots in the white part of the eye) occur during birth and are temporary and nothing to worry about.

3) A chemical irritation of the eye (red and swollen) may occur from the use of an antibiotic in the eyes at birth. Point out to the client and ask if the infant had eyedrops or ointment after birth. Ointment-caused irritation clears up in 2 to 5 days.

d. Birthmarks: There is usually no special care for birthmarks. The Home Health Aide should be aware of the most common birthmarks.

1) A port wine stain is a red/purple discoloration of the skin. The condition will have been noted by the physician/practitioner.

2) A stork beak mark consists of pale pink spots usually seen in the back of the neck and the eyelids.

3) A strawberry mark is a roundish raised mark of bright or dark red. It will have a rough surface.

4) Mongolian spots are dark blue or purple spots, irregular and bruiselike, seen mostly in the area right above the infant's buttocks. These are seen mostly in black infants.

e. Mouth

1) The normal newborn mouth has smooth, pink skin covering the lip surface. The inside of the cheeks, gums, and tongue should appear pink in color. Some infants' lips will develop crusts known as "sucking calluses" that will eventually be shed.

2) Thrush is seen as white or gray-white patches in the mouth or around the lips. Wipe ***very*** gently to determine that this is not milk. Wiping off thrush itself will cause the area to be left raw and bleeding. Notify the client of the suspicion of thrush so that the physician/practitioner may be consulted.

f. Extremities (arms and legs)

1) The extremities should be pinkish in color and may become mottled (lines of reddish color) or purplish when the infant is cold. Warm the baby and report to the client if color in the extremities remains purple after 15 minutes of warming.

2) Some infants may be born with problems of the hips that require special care. This should be noted in Homemaker's Plan of Care along with the client's instructions.

3) Extra fingers and toes may be seen in some infants. Note in the Homemaker's Plan of Care along with the client's instructions.

17. Explain the normal newborn's pattern for elimination.

a. Stools

1) Meconium consists of black, tarry stools passed after birth, changing to brownish green. At the fourth or fifth day, stools change according to the type of feeding.

(a) Human milk produces watery stools that may sometimes be light green.

(b) Cow's milk (formula) produces firmer stools than those of infants fed by human milk. These are passed usually one to three times a day. The color is yellow but not the bright yellow of breastfed infants.

2) Report to the client if no stools are passed for a day. Document the number of stools changed by you on the Homemaker's Progress Note. Document also if no stools are passed.

b. Voiding (urinating)

1) Six or more wet diapers in a 24-hour period show that the infant is getting enough fluids. The color of the urine should be pale yellow.

2) Report to the client if the infant has not wet in an 8-hour shift and inform the parent(s) that the physician/practitioner should be called.

MODULE 6: CARE OF THE PREGNANT AND POSTPARTUM WOMAN

This section covers the needs of the woman in the childbearing cycle. Upon completion of this unit, the learner should be prepared to accomplish the following.

1. Identify the objectives necessary to establish the woman's specific needs.
   a. Establish a "helping relationship" with the client and family (communication module).
   b. Complete the Plan of Care during the interview with the client and/or family.

2. Discuss prenatal growth and the baby's birth (modified from *The Expectant Woman's Guide*, Gerber Products Co., Fremont, MI, 1984.)

   Fertilization of the ovum by the sperm occurs in the fallopian tube, which is located on the topmost part of the uterus, deep in the woman's body. The sperm from the man are deposited in the vaginal canal and move toward the fallopian tube. When one successful sperm merges with the ovum, fertilization has occurred. The fertilized egg moves deeper into the uterine cavity and attaches to the uterine lining. There it forms a cluster of new cells that continue to grow rapidly to form the baby's body structure and organs. Inside the woman's body, the developing baby is protected and can move freely within the fluid-filled amniotic sac. During the 9 months of pregnancy, the placenta (a spongy sac) transmits nourishment and oxygen from the woman to the baby and disposes of wastes.

   Pregnancies may be divided into three 3-month stages, called trimesters. During each trimester, different things happen to both the woman's body and the growing baby. Changes occur in the size and shape of the uterus, abdomen, and breasts during pregnancy. During the first trimester, the uterus begins to stretch gently to make room for the growing embryo. The baby grows to a length of about 3 inches and a weight of 1 ounce by the end of the third month. It is during this time that the vital organs—heart, lungs, intestines, brain, eyes, ears, and skeleton—are formed.

   The baby grows to a length of about 14 inches and a weight of 2 pounds during the second trimester. Movements of the fetus, called "quickening," happen at around 20 weeks. The doctor will be able to hear the baby's heartbeat. Bones are growing, arm and leg joints are forming, and the baby's teeth are well started.

   During the final trimester, the baby's tissues and organs mature, and strength and weight are gained. The baby also starts kicking and moving about. The uterus moves higher in the abdomen until about the middle of the last month. The baby's head then begins to drop into the pelvis in preparation for delivery.

   Preparation-for-labor classes for expectant parents have played an important role in recent years. Experts give information on the development of the baby, body changes related to pregnancy, and what happens in labor. Each session includes tips on special breathing exercises that are helpful during delivery.

   Close to the time the baby will be born, the uterus gradually settles downward and forward. Mild, intermittent contractions as the muscles of the uterus tighten to push the baby down toward the vagina, and eventually out into the world, usually signal the start of labor. When the contractions come more often than every 10 minutes and last about 30 seconds, the doctor should be called. A small amount of pink discharge from the vagina is another sign of the start of labor. Once labor begins, no liquid or solid food should be taken.

   Labor may last between 6 and 12 hours for a woman's first baby. The first stage of labor is the dilating (expanding) and thinning out of the cervix (the narrow opening to the uterus) to allow the baby's head to pass through. The contractions gradually intensify as this thinning occurs. If the membranes have not broken by the time the cervix has expanded about two inches, the doctor may break them.

When the cervix is fully dilated, the next stage of labor, the delivery, begins. The contractions should come every 2 to 3 minutes. Slowly, during a contraction, the baby's head emerges with the face turned downward. Gradually the head rotates as the shoulders, abdomen, and legs follow rapidly. Then, the remaining fluid in the uterus is expelled.

The last stage of labor is the delivery of the placenta or afterbirth. The type of care given to the baby right after birth depends on where the baby is born. Many hospitals let women breastfeed their newborn babies immediately. Other hospitals follow a more traditional routine, which includes some separation of the woman and the baby after birth. The doctor can discuss these options with the woman early in her pregnancy.

During the first few weeks after the baby is born, the uterus starts to return to its prepregnancy size. This process is usually faster in breastfeeding women. Simple exercises done with a doctor's approval will help tone stomach and abdominal muscles. Most doctors like to give the new mother a physical checkup about 6 weeks after delivery. Menstruation usually returns within 3 to 10 weeks after delivery in non-nursing women. In most nursing women, it may be longer before menstruation returns.

3. Identify the normal discomforts of pregnancy, the physiological basis for the discomfort, management of the discomfort, and indications of potential problems that should be reported to the Home Care Supervisor.

   a. Backache

      1) Definition: Nonpathological lumbosacral backache usually occurring in the second and third trimesters.

      2) Physiological basis

         (a) The increased size of the uterus contributes to muscle strain.

         (b) Changes in posture also contribute to muscle strain.

         (c) Excessive bending, walking, and lifting are other causes of backache.

         (d) High back pain can occur from the increasing size of the breasts.

      3) Management of high back pain

         (a) Suggest a supportive bra.

         (b) Client can stretch her arms over her head to exercise the muscles of the upper back.

      4) Management of lower back pain

         (a) Encourage good posture and body alignment.

         (b) Teach proper body mechanics.

         (c) Encourage the client to wear low-heeled shoes.

         (d) Exercise as permitted by the obstetrics (OB) care provider.

         (e) Place pillows in a manner that will position and straighten out the back, alleviating pulling and strain.

         (f) Relief measures include moist warm compresses and massage.

         (g) Acetaminophen will help, if permitted by the OB care provider. Caution the client against taking any medications without the OB care provider's knowledge.

         (h) Observe the client to rule out preterm labor or infection, especially a urinary tract infection or kidney infection.

5) Indicators to refer the client to your supervisor.
   (a) Severe persistent pain should be reported to the Home Care Supervisor.
   (b) Signs and symptoms of premature labor or urinary tract infection should also be reported.

b. Braxton Hicks contractions
   1) Definition: Uterine contractions not associated with labor, felt in the second and third trimesters. They are usually infrequent and irregular in timing.
   2) Physiological basis: The exact mechanism is unknown but is thought to be related to hormonal preparation of the uterus for labor.
   3) Management
      (a) Determine the frequency and duration of the contractions.
      (b) Encourage the client to rest on her side.
      (c) Advise deep, relaxing breathing.
   4) Indicators to refer the client to your supervisor.
      (a) Contractions coming with any regular frequency or occurring within 20 minutes of each other should be reported to your supervisor.
      (b) Severe pain should be referred to your supervisor.
      (c) Any gush or leaking of fluid from the vagina is an indication that the supervisor should be called.
      (d) Blood showing in vaginal secretions should be referred to your supervisor.
      (e) Burning or pain during urination need to be discussed as well.

c. Constipation
   1) Definition: Hard, infrequent stools; may occur throughout pregnancy.
   2) Physiological basis
      (a) The smooth muscle of the bowel relaxes due to increased progesterone.
      (b) Increased absorption of water from the bowel contributes to hard stool.
      (c) The bowels are compressed by the enlarged uterus.
      (d) Iron supplements can also lead to constipation.
      (e) Decreased activity is another contributor.
   3) Management
      (a) The client should drink 8 to 10 glasses of water each day.
      (b) Encourage daily exercise, as permitted by the OB care provider.
      (c) Increase roughage foods in the client's diet, e.g., apples, salads, whole wheat and bran cereals, and prunes.
      (d) Use stool softeners only as prescribed by the OB care provider.
   4) Notify your supervisor if the client complains of severe discomfort.

d. Dizziness/fainting
   1) Definition: Lightheadedness, dizzy or spinning feeling, loss of consciousness; occurs more frequently in the first and third trimesters.

2) Physiological basis
   (a) Changes in circulation as a result of pregnancy lead to dizziness.
   (b) Sudden standing causes blood to pool in lower extremities.
   (c) Hypotension is another factor contributing to this problem.
   (d) Low blood sugar, hyperventilation, or anemia also cause dizziness.
3) Management
   (a) Encourage the client to rise slowly when she stands up.
   (b) Encourage her to lie on her side to improve circulation.
   (c) Suggest small, frequent meals.
   (d) Advise slow, deep breathing.
   (e) Determine from the client or supervisor whether the client suffers from anemia; if so, encourage the client to eat foods high in iron. If the OB care provider has prescribed iron, remind the client to take her medication.
4) Indicators to refer the client to your supervisor.
   (a) Loss of consciousness should be reported to your supervisor.
   (b) Notify your supervisor if the client's blood pressure rises more than 30 systolic or 15 diastolic.
   (c) A persistent headache should also be investigated.
   (d) Complaints of reduced fetal activity are worthy of report to your supervisor.

e. Edema
   1) Definition: Edema is swelling in the extremities, usually developing in the second and third trimesters.
   2) Physiological basis
      (a) Increased blood volume causes swelling of the extremities.
      (b) The enlarged uterus causes impaired return circulation in the lower extremities.
      (c) Increased hormones result in increased sodium and water retention.
   3) Management
      (a) Take the client's blood pressure to determine the signs and symptoms of preeclampsia.
      (b) The client should avoid restrictive clothing.
      (c) Elevate the client's legs, whenever possible, above the level of the heart.
      (d) The client should rest lying on her side to improve return circulation to the heart.
      (e) Support hose will also help with edema.
      (f) Advise drinking 8 to 10 glasses of water each day.
   4) Indicators to refer the client to your supervisor: Increases in baseline blood pressure of more than 30 systolic or 15 diastolic and/or facial edema indicate potential preeclampsia.

f. Frequent urination and nocturia

1) Definition: Frequent passage of urine and increased night urination occurring in the first and third trimesters.
2) Physiological basis
   (a) The enlarging uterus places increased pressure on the bladder.
   (b) The bladder has less room to expand and thus has less capacity.
   (c) Urine production increases at night.
3) Management
   (a) Encourage the client to practice kegel exercises.
   (b) Limit her fluid intake at night.
   (c) Advise frequent urination to help prevent urinary tract infection, a frequent problem during pregnancy that can lead to premature labor.
   (d) Determine if the client has signs and symptoms of infection by assessing her vital signs and determining if there is any pain during urination.
4) Indicators to refer the client to your supervisor: Report any suspicion of urinary tract infection, diabetes, or ruptured membranes to your supervisor.

g. Heartburn/indigestion
   1) Definition: Condition characterized by a reflux of gastric acid into the esophagus.
   2) Physiological basis
      (a) Intolerance to fatty food causes heartburn and indigestion.
      (b) Increased progesterone relaxes the cardiac sphincter.
      (c) The enlarging uterus compresses the stomach.
   3) Management
      (a) Smaller, more frequent meals will help.
      (b) The client should also decrease her consumption of fatty foods.
      (c) The client should avoid lying down after meals.
      (d) Dry crackers and teas such as chamomile, comfrey, and peppermint will help alleviate the discomfort.
   4) Indicators to refer the client to your supervisor.
      (a) Persistent, severe symptoms should be reported to your supervisor.
      (b) You should notify your supervisor in cases of pain, vomiting, and fever.

h. Hemorrhoids
   1) Definition: Swelling of veins in and around the anus.
   2) Physiological basis
      (a) The enlarging uterus creates circulatory congestion.
      (b) Constipation is a contributing factor.
      (c) Increased progesterone relaxes the walls of the veins.
   3) Management
      (a) Avoid constipation and straining with bowel movements.

(b) Encourage the client to practice kegel exercises.

(c) Advise sitz baths.

(d) Adequate rest, and exercise as permitted by the OB care provider, will help also.

(e) Ice the area.

(f) The client should rest in bed with her hips and lower extremities elevated.

(g) Analgesic ointments may be prescribed by the OB care provider.

4) Indicators to refer the client to your supervisor.

(a) Severe, persistent symptoms should be reported.

(b) Bleeding, swelling, and severe pain are all reasons to contact your supervisor.

4. Identify the most common conditions associated with premature birth. (The instructor should refer to the textbook resources to discuss each condition in depth.)
   a. Premature labor contractions
   b. Hypertensive disorders
   c. Diabetes

5. Identify danger signs in pregnancy that require the immediate attention of the OB care provider.
   a. Regular contractions with or without pain for over 1 hour before the 37th week of gestation
   b. Rupture of amniotic fluid before the 37th week of gestation
   c. Appearance of bloody show before the 37th week of gestation
   d. Frank vaginal bleeding at any time
   e. Illness: Any fever, vomiting, diarrhea, headache, blurred vision, or chills
   f. Seizures usually associated with eclampsia in pregnancy: Preeclampsia, progression of proteinuria, hypertension with an increase in basal blood pressure of more than 30 systolic and 15 diastolic, and edema
   g. Reduction in usual fetal movement
   h. Foul-smelling vaginal discharge
   i. Abdominal pain

6. Identify anatomical changes in the postpartum woman.
   a. Return of blood volume to prepregnant state.
      1) The blood volume of the pregnant woman increases by at least 40% to allow her to tolerate the blood loss of delivery.
      2) Many women lose 300 to 400 ml (a little less than $^1/_2$ quart) of blood.
      3) Due to increased blood clotting factors in the blood, encourage ambulation to prevent blood clotting problems.
   b. Genital tract
      1) The cervix may be bruised and have some small lacerations.

2) At birth, the uterus weighs 11 times its prepregnant weight; afterward, it rapidly shrinks back into the pelvis (2.2 pounds after delivery reduces 11 to 12 ounces 2 weeks after delivery).

3) Uterine size is slightly increased after each pregnancy.

4) Vaginal structures may be bruised, sore, and swollen due to birth trauma, episiotomy, and/or lacerations.

5) The client will experience "bleeding" consisting of blood tissue and mucus for about 2 weeks. It is heaviest in the first 2 days after delivery and should decrease after this.

c. Urinary tract

1) Increased urination should begin within 12 hours after delivery to allow for elimination of excess tissue fluid accumulated in pregnancy.

2) Pelvic soreness due to labor, vaginal lacerations, or episiotomy may be reduced after voiding.

d. Gastrointestinal tract

1) Bowel movements may be delayed for several days because of decreased muscle tone in intestines, prelabor diarrhea, lack of food, dehydration, and/or tenderness of the genital structures.

2) For some women, bowel habits must be reestablished through special attention to diet and fluid intake.

e. Breasts

1) Considerable enlargement of the breasts occurs during pregnancy in response to changes in hormones.

2) The size of the milk ducts increases during pregnancy, and by the sixth or seventh month small amounts of "pre-milk," colostrum, may be expressed from the nipple.

3) Two to 3 days after delivery, a surge of actual milk may be expected.

4) Infant suckling causes stimulation that results in increased hormone production. Production of hormone causes the milk ducts to contract and "let down" milk.

f. Abdomen

1) The muscles of the abdomen are stretched; the client will have been instructed by her physician/practitioner/nurse as to when exercises may be started.

2) Abdominal cesarean section

(a) The classical type involves a vertical incision (up and down).

(b) A transverse incision runs across the top of the pubic hairline ("bikini" incision).

7. Explain the types of episiotomy.

a. A median episiotomy is the most common and generally the least painful. Occasionally there may be an extension through the rectal sphincter (third-degree laceration) or even into the anal canal (fourth-degree laceration).

b. With a mediolateral episiotomy, third-degree lacerations may occur but fourth-degree lacerations may be avoided. The blood loss is greater, repair is more difficult and painful, and there is usually more pain during healing.

8. Identify the daily dietary allowances of nonpregnant, pregnant, and breastfeeding females. (See Table 3-1.)

9. Identify the recommended number of food group servings. (See Table 3-2.)

10. Discuss specific types of food and food preparation in relation to the postpartum woman.
    a. Determine from the client if her physician/practitioner has recommended a special diet.
    b. She should drink 8 to 12 glasses of water daily (average 10).
    c. Also advise her to consume plenty of protein, fresh vegetables, fresh fruit, and milk.
    d. Bran cereals or dried fruits prevent constipation. (Cesarean section clients and clients with fourth-degree lacerations may have received instructions to avoid roughage foods; check with the client.)
    e. Cesarean section clients may have discomfort due to "gas pain." If acceptable to the client, 1 tablespoon of dark molasses three times a day will help the intestines move sooner and push out the gas. This may be mixed in water, juice, tea, or milk or may be taken by itself.
    f. Avoid "gassy" foods for all postpartum clients (broccoli, cauliflower, baked beans, fried foods, hot dogs, and cucumbers).

11. Identify the nutritional needs of the pregnant teen and problems interfering with their compliance.
    a. Adolescence (13 to 18 years) has special nutritional needs unrelated to pregnancy because of rapid growth and development of the body.
    b. Adolescence represents a time when the diet may not be closely supervised by parents and "junk food" becomes the mainstay of the diet.
    c. One in 10 adolescents who become pregnant is obese. The fat-conscious teen may have not been getting adequate nutrition.
    d. Underweight adolescents are more prone to anemia (iron-poor blood), bone problems, and infections.
    e. Caloric requirements—to be provided by nutritional foods—for the pregnant and breastfeeding teen
        1) 11 to 14 years
            (a) Pregnancy: 2,700 calories
            (b) Breastfeeding: 2,900 calories
        2) 15 to 18 years
            (a) Pregnancy: 2,400 calories
            (b) Breastfeeding: 2,600 calories
    f. Be aware to ask the client if her physician/practitioner has discussed the WIC Program (special Supplemental Food Program for Women and Children). If not, instruct client to discuss with physician/practitioner.

12. Discuss dietary habits and acceptable foods with the pregnant/postpartum woman. Refer to Box 3-3. (From S.J. Reeder, L. Martin, D. Koniak-Griffin. *Maternity Nursing: Family, Newborn, and Women's Health, 18th ed.* Lippincott–Raven, 1997.)

TABLE 3-1
Daily Dietary Allowances of Nonpregnant, Lactating, and Pregnant Females[1]

	Nonpregnant[2] (years of age)						Lactating (mos)	
	11–14	15–18	19–24	25–50	51+[1]	Pregnant	1–6	7–12
Protein (g)	46	44	46	50	50	60	65	62
Vitamin A (m g RE)[3]	800	800	800	800	800	800	1300	1200
Vitamin D (m g)[3]	10	10	10	5	5	10	10	10
Vitamin E (mg a-TE)[3]	8	8	8	8	8	10	12	11
Vitamin K (m g)	45	55	60	65	65	65	65	65
Vitamin C (mg)	50	60	60	60	60	70	95	90
Thiamin (mg)	1.1	1.1	1.1	1.1	1.0	1.5	1.6	1.6
Riboflavin (mg)	1.3	1.3	1.3	1.3	1.2	1.6	1.8	1.7
Niacin (mg NE)[3]	15	15	15	15	13	17	20	20
Vitamin B_6 (mg)	1.4	1.5	1.6	1.6	1.6	2.2	2.1	2.1
Folate (m g)	150	180	180	180	180	400	280	260
Vitamin B_{12} (m g)	2.0	2.0	2.0	2.0	2.0	2.2	2.6	2.6
Calcium (mg)	1200	1200	1200	800	800	1200	1200	1200
Phosphorus (mg)	1200	1200	1200	800	800	1200	1200	1200
Magnesium (mg)	280	300	280	280	280	300	355	340
Iron (mg)	15	15	15	15	10	30	15	15
Zinc (mg)	12	12	12	12	12	15	19	16
Iodine (m g)	150	150	150	150	150	175	200	200
Selenium (m g)	45	50	55	55	55	65	75	75

[1]From Food and Nutrition Board, 1989, Recommended dietary allowances. National Academy of Sciences—National Research Council, Washington, D.C.

[2]Heights and weights: 11–14 years: weight 46 kg (101 pounds), height 157 cm (62 inches); 15–18 years: weight 55 kg (120 pounds), height 163 cm (64 inches); 19–24 years: weight 58 kg (128 pounds), height 164 cm (65 inches); 25–50 years: weight 63 kg (138 pounds), height 163 cm (64 inches); 51+ years: weight 65 kg (143 pounds), height 160 cm (63 inches). These figures are based on actual medians in the USA; they are not meant to indicate ideal height:weight ratios.

[3]Vitamin A is expressed as retinol equivalents; 1 m g RE = 1 m g retinol or 6 m g β-carotene. Vitamin D is expressed as cholecalciferol;
10 m g cholecalciferol = 400 IU vitamin D. Vitamin E is expressed as α-tocopherol equivalents; 1 mg α-TE = 1 mg d-α-toco-

TABLE 3-2.
Daily Food Guide for Women

	Minimum Number of Servings		
Food Group	Nonpregnant Adult Woman	Nonpregnant Adult Woman	Pregnant/Lactating/Adolescent Adult Woman
Protein foods	5*	5*	7*
Milk products	3	2	3
Breads, cereal grains	7**	6**	7**
Fruits and vegetables			
Vitamin C-rich	1	1	1
Vitamin A-rich	1	1	1
Other	3	3	3

*Each serving is equivalent to 1 oz. of animal protein; at least one serving should be from the vegetable protein list (two servings during pregnancy or lactation).

**At least four servings should be from whole grains.

California Department of Health Service, MCH/WIC (1990).

BOX 3-3: NUTRITIONAL TEACHING GUIDES

Food Group	One Serving Equals		Recommended Minimum Servings: Male/non-pregnant female	Recommended Minimum Servings: Pregnant/breast-feeding
PROTEIN FOODS Excellent sources of protein, vitamin B_6, iron, and zinc. Animal protein supplies vitamin B_{12}. Vegetable protein is a good source of folic acid, magnesium, and fiber.	ANIMAL PROTEIN: 1 oz cooked lean meat, fish, poultry, or seafood 1 egg 2 hot dogs 2 slices luncheon meat 2 oz or 3 links sausage 2 fish sticks	VEGETABLE PROTEIN: 1/2 cup cooked dry beans 3 oz tofu 1 oz or 1/4 cup peanuts, pumpkin, or sunflower seeds 1 1/2 oz or 1/3 cup other nuts 2 tbsp peanut butter	5 Have at least 1 serving from vegetable protein	7
MILK PRODUCTS* Excellent sources of protein and calcium. In addition, milk products are good sources of vitamins A, B_{12}, riboflavin, and zinc. Fortified fluid milk contains 100 IU of vitamin D per cup.	1 cup milk or yogurt 1 cup milkshake 1 1/2 cups cream soups (made with milk) 1 1/2 oz or 1/3 cup grated brick-type cheese (like cheddar or jack)	1 1/2 slices presliced American cheese 4 tbsp parmesan 2 cups cottage cheese 1 cup pudding or custard 1 1/2 cups ice cream or frozen yogurt	2 (3 for teens)	3
BREADS, CEREALS, GRAINS All provide carbohydrates and some protein, as well as thiamine, riboflavin, niacin, and iron. Whole grains provide additional vitamin B_6, folic acid, vitamin E, magnesium, zinc, and fiber.	1 slice bread 1 dinner roll 1/2 bun, bagel, English muffin or pita 1 small tortilla 1/4 cup dry cereal 1/2 cup granola	1/2 cup cooked cereal, noodles, or rice 4 tbsp wheat germ 1 4-in pancake or waffle 1 muffin 8 medium crackers 4 graham cracker squares	6 Have at least 4 servings from whole-grain products	7
VITAMIN C-RICH FRUITS AND VEGETABLES Excellent sources of vitamin C and fiber. They also supply vitamins A, B_6, and folic acid.	6 oz orange, grapefruit, tomato, vegetable juice coctail or fruit juice enriched with vitamin C 1 orange, kiwi, mango 1/2 grapefruit, cantaloupe 1/4 papaya 2 tangerines, tomatoes	1/2 cup strawberries, broccoli, brussels sprouts, cabbage, cauliflower, snow peas, sweet peppers, or tomato puree 2 tbsp fresh or 1/2 cup cooked hot peppers	1	1

*See Nondairy Calicum-Rich Foods below.

BOX 3-3: *(continued)*

Food Group	One Serving Equals		Recommended Minimum Servings: Male/non-pregnant female	Recommended Minimum Servings: Pregnant/breast-feeding
VITAMIN A-RICH FRUITS AND VEGETABLES Excellent sources of beta-carotene and vitamin A. Most are good sources of fiber. The dark green vegetables also supply good amounts of vitamin B_6, folic acid, and magnesium.	6 oz apricot nectar or vegetable juice cocktail 3 raw or 1/4 cup dried apricots 1/4 cantaloupe or mango 1/2 papaya 1 small or 1/2 cup sliced carrots	1/2 cup greens (beet, chard, collards, dandelion, kale, mustard, spinach) 1/2 cup pumpkin, sweet potato or winter squash 2 tbsp raw or cooked hot peppers 2 tomatoes	1	1
OTHER FRUITS AND VEGETABLES Provide carbohydrates and fiber as well as smaller amounts of other essential vitamins and minerals.	6 oz fruit juice 1 medium or 1/2 cup sliced fruit (apple, banana, berries, cherries, grapes, peach, pear) 1/2 cup pineapple or watermelon 1/2 cup dried fruit	1/2 cup sliced vegetable (asparagus, beets, green beans, celery, corn, eggplant, mushrooms, onion, peas, potato, summer squash) 1/2 artichoke 1 cup lettuce	3	3

FOLIC ACID-RICH FOODS

These foods are rich in folic acid, a B- vitamin especially important during pregnancy because of its role in growth and repair. Pregnant women should have at least four servings daily of these foods.

PROTEIN FOODS

Beans: baked, garbanzo, kidney, navy, pinto, pork'n'beans	Peanuts
Lentils	Split peas
Liver	Sunflower seeds
	Yeast, nutritional

FRUITS AND VEGETABLES

Asparagus	Lettuce: bibb, Boston endive, romaine

NONDAIRY CALCIUM-RICH FOODS

Each of the following is approximately equivalent in calcium to one serving from the milk products group (250–300 mg calcium):

Almonds	4 oz
Beans: baked, pork'n'beans	2 cups
Broccoli, fresh cooked	1 1/2 cups
Greens: turnip, cooked	1 1/2 cups
Greens: bok choy, collard, dandelion, cooked	2 cups
Greens: kale, mustard, cooked	3 cups
Molasses, blackstrap	2 tbsp
Oranges	5 medium
Salmon (with bones)	1/2 cup canned

13. Identify the specific needs for rest in the postpartum woman.
    a. The client needs the opportunity to obtain plenty of rest.
    b. Activity should be limited to care of herself and her baby.
    c. Assistance should be obtained to take care of siblings, meals, laundry, and household duties for at least 1 week for the woman who has delivered her child vaginally and 3 to 4 weeks for the woman who has delivered by cesarean section.
    d. Fatigue decreases the breast milk supply and the ability to deal with changes and new responsibilities.

14. Identify the role of ambulation (walking) during the woman's recovery.
    a. Most clients without complications will have been instructed to have short, frequent periods of ambulation. Early walking has been shown to be instrumental in reducing the incidence of blood clotting (thrombosis) and helps greatly in rapid recovery of strength.
    b. Clients having a vaginal delivery should attempt to stay on one floor for a week, or to limit stair climbing to once or twice a day; stairs should be taken slowly. Assist the client in accomplishing this goal.
    c. Clients having a cesarean birth will usually be strongly advised to stay on one floor and to go up and down stairs just once a day after the first week. Assist the client in accomplishing this goal.

15. Describe suggested breastfeeding techniques.
    a. Wash your hands.
    b. Assist the mother to assume a comfortable position. For the woman who has delivered her baby by cesarean section, this may mean lying on her side with a pillow to protect the incision for the first few days.
    c. Encourage the mother to help the baby start nursing by holding him or her close so that the baby's cheek touches the breast.
    d. The baby should take as much of the areola (the darker area surrounding the nipple) as possible into his or her mouth, not just the nipple. The nipple should be erect; the mother may need to roll an inverted nipple between her thumb and index finger to make it protrude.
    e. If the mother's breast is full, explain to her that using one finger to press the breast away from the infant's nose will allow easier breathing for the baby.
    f. Encourage the mother to use both breasts and to alternate the side she begins with; a safety pin fastened to the bra strap may help to remind her.
    g. Never pull the nipple from the baby's mouth. To break suction, press the breast away from the corner of the mouth or lift the baby's lip by putting a clean finger into the corner of the mouth.
    h. The baby should be burped after feedings.
    i. A nursing bra may provide comfortable support.
    j. Encourage the mother to leave the nursing flaps of her bra down whenever possible to allow the nipples to dry. Allow the nipples to dry before applying any cream recommended by the physician/practitioner.
    k. The mother may ask questions about cramping during nursing. This is nature's way of returning the uterus to its normal size.

l. Breastfed babies may desire nursing every 2 to 3 hours.

m. The mother's milk supply will increase with an increased amount of nursing.

n. Do not use soap or antiseptics on the nipples as they tend to cause excessive drying of the skin.

o. Encourage the mother to drink 10 glasses of water daily to help keep her supply of milk adequate, and to avoid caffeine and tobacco. Caffeine and nicotine eventually enter the mother's milk and are consumed by the baby.

p. Six or more wet diapers a day assures the mother that her baby is getting enough milk.

16. Discuss problems of sore nipples and some usual comfort measures to ease the pain.

a. Nipples may be red or cracked and may even bleed.

1) This may be normal as the nipples become accustomed to infant's sucking.

2) Other causes may be poor positioning, pull on nipples, taking baby off breast incorrectly, incomplete air drying of nipples after feeding, and irritating chemicals or objects, such as soap, shampoo, strong laundry detergent, rough clothing, or plastic liners against nipples.

b. Comfort measures to suggest to the client.

1) Rotate positions in which the baby feeds so that the infant does not constantly clamp down on same sore area.

2) Start feeding on the less sore nipple; the infant sucks the hardest in the first 10 minutes.

3) The large portion of the nipple should be in the baby's mouth, not just the tip.

4) Suction should always be broken before removing the infant from the breast.

5) Eucerin cream may be recommended to clients because it is a mineral oil-based cream and has no preservatives or alcohol. The client may have other instructions from the physician/practitioner and should consult with that person before changing.

6) Warm salt water soaks may be ordered by the physician/practitioner.

(a) Boil 1 quart of water with 1/2 teaspoon of salt for 10 minutes. (Tap water contains germs that may contribute to breast infection.)

(b) Allow to cool for 1/2 hour.

(c) Wash your hands according to standard handwashing procedures.

(d) Test the water with your finger; it should not be hot. Do not use until the water is lukewarm.

(e) Wash your hands at all times before testing the water.

(f) Locate household items that may be used as a compress; peripads are excellent, and washcloths, etc. may be used.

(g) Locate a plastic covering: plastic wrap, plastic bags, etc.

(h) Wash your hands according to standard handwashing procedure.

(i) Take the sterile salt water, compress, and plastic to the client.

(j) The client may wish to apply the salt water compresses herself; she should wash her hands first. If assistance is requested, wash your hands, dip the compresses in water, gently apply to nipples, and cover with the plastic to prevent heat loss. Take care to ask the client if the compresses are too warm.

(k) The skin should be checked in 5 minutes to make sure the compresses are not too warm.

7) Apply ice to the nipple before feeding.

8) Use a nipple shield.

9) Some physicians/practitioners will recommend the use of tea bags on the nipples; tea bags may be saved from a cup of tea, but wash hands well before handling anything that will have contact with nipples.

17. Explain the problems and solutions of engorged breasts.

a. Clients will experience fullness and heaviness on the second to third day postpartum when the milk comes in.

b. Milk may become "plugged up" and the breast and nipple will appear shiny and hard.

c. The infant may have trouble attaching to the breast because of this fullness. The client can express a small amount before feeding if this occurs.

d. The client should be encouraged to nurse on both breasts at each feeding.

e. Warm compresses to the upper area of the breasts, warm showers, massage, and hand expression may relieve the fullness.

f. The client's bra should fit well, not cutting or binding her skin (evidenced by redness of skin along the bra lines).

18. Discuss proper methods of breast pumping and milk storage.

a. Breast massage and hand expression: These techniques may be used before feeding to bring the milk down to the baby, to relieve postpartum fullness, and before pumping or hand expressing to decrease the time spent on collection.

1) To massage, place one hand under breast; with the other hand, starting from the shoulder, stroke down toward the nipple. Also stroke under the breast and then up. Continue for 1 minute.

2) To hand express, put the thumb and forefinger on areola about 1 inch back from the nipple. Press back toward the chest and squeeze together to compress the milk duct.

b. Use of mechanical breast pump

1) Egnell Electric Breast Pump

(a) There are two purposes for using a breast pump: to stimulate the formation of breast milk in the woman who is unable to nurse her baby and to maintain an existing supply of breast milk in the woman who must temporarily stop breastfeeding her baby.

(b) Remember, the Egnell is very efficient as a breast pump but is neither as efficient nor as gentle as the baby nursing. Therefore, the pumping schedule should be followed as written. The pumping woman should be instructed in the care of her nipples, especially proper airing and use of Eucerin cream.

The woman should be instructed to pump at regular intervals to establish a pumping routine of every 3 hours, or 2 hours if the breasts need to be emptied. (Encourage milk let-down with warm compresses and by massaging the breast toward the nipple before applying pump.) Remember that pumping is easily put off because there is no baby crying to be nursed. However, stress that keeping to a regular pumping routine will establish a milk supply and enable the woman to give her baby her breast milk.

Cracked, sore, or bleeding nipples can occur with pumping, as with nursing. These normal problems of nursing are treated the same way as with a nursing woman. The woman should be taught to air her nipples well after each pumping session and to use a small dot of Eucerin cream massaged into sore nipples. If slight bleeding occurs from cracked nipples, the milk may still be used for the baby. The sore, cracked, bleeding nipples will heal in a few days with proper care. Eucerin cream need not be removed.

(c) Pumping schedule: Pump each breast the scheduled amount of time at each session. (See Table 3-3.) Continue at this level for the rest of the pumping time. If needed, pump more frequently but not longer.

Both breasts must be pumped twice at each pumping session. This ensures a more adequate emptying of the milk ducts and is easier on the nipples.

The woman should be told to pump her breasts every 3 hours by the clock. She should pump once during the night if she awakens or is uncomfortable. The obtained milk is poured into a sterile bottle labeled with the name, date, and time and refrigerated. The refrigerated milk may be kept for 24 hours. If not used, it should be discarded. Once warmed for use, the milk must be used at that feeding or discarded.

The woman who has already been nursing her baby and must temporarily stop nursing may begin pumping at the day number 4 level and maintain it until finished with pumping. She may pump at intervals as needed to relieve her filling breasts, every hour if needed. She must pump during the night to prevent overfilling of her breasts.

If the client is sending her milk to her hospitalized infant: Every intensive care nursery has different procedures for storing the breast milk. Some hospitals want refrigerated milk, other frozen. Some hospitals want milk collected in glass containers, others in plastic. Have the woman or nurse call the intensive care nursery and get specific instructions for the storage and collection of breast milk. Put this information in your Plan of Care notes.

(d) Assembly of Egnell Electric Breast Pump

- Review the manufacturer's directions for use.
- Press the breast shield lid unit on top of the milk bottle until it snaps in place.
- To remove the lid, hold the milk bottle firmly with both hands and push the lid upward with both thumbs.
- Connect the tubing from the pump.
- Place the preassembled safety overflow bottle in the small recess provided for it in the pump.

TABLE 3-3.
Breast Pumping Schedule

	Right Breast	Left Breast	Right Breast	Left Breast
Day 1	2 min	2 min	2 min	2 min
Day 2	3 min	3 min	3 min	3 min
Day 3	4 min	4 min	4 min	4 min
Day 4	5 min	5min	5 min	5 min

- Place the bottle retainer over the safety overflow bottle lid so it fits snugly into the grooves and tighten the thumb screw.
- Connect the plastic tubing supplied in the kit to the pipe in the safety overflow bottle underneath the arrow (pipe connection).
- Connect the other end of this tube to the pipe extending from the breast shield lid attached to the milk bottle.
- Connect the remaining tube from the breast pump to the remaining protrusion on the lid of the overflow bottle.
- ***The tubing must be connected properly or the overflow milk can go directly into the pump***.
- Connect the electric cord from the pump to the grounded wall outlet.
- The pump is now ready to be used.

(e) Operation of the Egnell Electric Breast Pump

- Establish a convenient place to pump.
- Place the pump on a table in a convenient spot.
- Have a large glass of something to drink within easy reach. Drink only until thirst is quenched.
- Have a clean towel available for use if necessary.
- Have the woman sit in a comfortable chair or upright in bed, sitting straight up or leaning slightly forward. (It is important that she not be lying down because it is possible to get milk backup into the pump this way.)

(f) Adjusting suction

- Always start on minimum suction even when changing from one breast to another.
- Move the regulator toward "normal" suction according to nipple comfort level.
- The pump operates best when the regulator is set at "normal" suction. For very sore or cracked nipples, the pump should be used at the minimum setting only.

(g) Choosing the proper breast shield unit

- If breast and nipples are small to medium, use a normal size breast shield. If breast and nipples are large, use a large size breast shield.
- Place the shield over the nipple before starting the pump. (Lubricate the shield with colostrum or sterile water.)
- Keep the shield pressed against the breast so that a seal is formed.
- To remove the shield, turn off the pump and stop pressing; the shield will release from the breast.

(h) Use of the milk bottle: The milk bottle should be filled no more than 2/3 full. Keep the bottle steady and in an upright position; otherwise, milk may be sucked into the overflow safety bottle.

(i) Use of the overflow safety bottle: If milk should go into the overflow safety bottle, switch off the pump at once. Discard the entire kit and get a new one.

(j) Care of Egnell Electric Breast Pump equipment

- The pump exterior must be cleaned weekly with household disinfectant cleaner.
- If milk spillage occurs involving the pump and/or cart, cleaning must be done immediately.

(k) Milk collection set-up

- The kit includes collection bottle and breast shield with lid, plastic milk bottle, overflow safety bottle, and plastic tubing. Two breast shield/lid combinations are available, either large or normal size.
- A sterile set-up is obtained for each woman; the set-up is washed with mild soap and rinsed in hot water after each pumping session.
- Both breasts are pumped with the same set-up, thereby collecting all the milk into one bottle.
- Collected milk is transferred to an empty sterile water bottle labeled with the woman's name, date, and time of collection.
- Milk is promptly stored in refrigerator or freezer as required.

(l) Connecting tubing: Connects the collecting set-up with the small overflow bottle.

- If tubing is contaminated with milk overflow, it must be changed immediately.
- Tubing does not need to be sterile (tubing cannot be autoclaved).

(m) Small overflow bottle protects pump in case of milk overflow. The overflow bottle needs to be changed only if accidental overflow occurs. This is to be done immediately; check manufacturer's instructions. Notify Home Care Supervisor immediately.

(n) Document all actions in Home Health Aide's Progress Notes.

2) Kaneson Breast Pump

(a) Used to relieve postpartum engorgement or for the woman to pump breast milk for the baby who is unable to nurse.

(b) Parts: 1 plastic flange, 1 plastic bottle (flange fits inside bottle; 1 rubber gasket (on flange), 2 plastic nipple adaptors, 1 plastic cover, 1 rubber nipple, 1 bottle brush, 2 extra rubber gaskets.

(c) Procedure for pumping

- The woman should wash her hands and do breast massage and hand expression.
- If the milk is not in yet, warm compresses may be used in addition to massage before pumping.
- Place plastic flange inside the plastic bottle. Place nipple adapter in flange as necessary.
- Lubricate plastic flange with sterile water or breast milk.
- Place pump on nipple slightly off center.
- Pull pump out as far as comfortable, allowing milk to flow.
- Push in pump and pull out again, repeating process.
- Pump 3 to 5 minutes per side, rotating back and forth as necessary.

- If milk is to be frozen, chill and freeze as soon as possible (chilled milk may be layered in a frozen bottle; collect 3 1/2 ounces in a 4-ounce bottle.)

(d) Procedure for cleaning

- Disassemble pump-flange and bottle (do not remove rubber gasket).
- Wash with household disinfectant.
- Double wrap and date pieces and autoclave.
- No need to autoclave nipple, battle brush, and extra gaskets. Keep these in box.

3) Reasons for pumping and type of pump to use

(a) There are several pumps available, ranging in price and effectiveness. Naval, Evenflo, and Kaneson are hand pumps; Medela, Egnell, and Neonatal Axicare are electric pumps. (See breast pump information sheet.)

(b) Some mothers prefer to collect breast milk by pumping.

(c) Some mothers must be separated from their infants. They should probably use an electric, Lopuco, or Kaneson type pump. These women should be referred to a Premature and High Risk Counselor.

(d) Some mothers pump to go back to work or school or for an occasional bottle. They could use a Lopuco or Kaneson type pump and should be referred to a regular nursing women's group.

c. Collection by milk cups

1) A milk cup is a plastic device that fits over the breast with an opening in the center for the nipple. The milk cup should be sterilized before use, then placed over the breast with the small hole on the upper side. The collected milk can then be poured into a sterile container for storage.

2) Some woman leak from one breast while nursing from the other. By using a plastic milk cup on the leaking breast, the woman can easily collect milk that would otherwise be lost.

3) Other uses include drawing out inverted nipples or relieving postpartum fullness. The milk cup should be worn 1/2 hour before feeding for these purposes.

d. Collection and storage of breast milk

1) Milk may be collected and stored by mothers who wish their babies to have breast milk in a bottle. It can be collected by hand expression, milk cups, or breast pump. A collection may produce only 1 ounce, so the mother should start ahead of time.

2) Milk should be collected in a sterile (boiled for 5 minutes) container.

3) Milk should be chilled and then frozen. Milk may be layered in a frozen bottle. Pour only chilled milk on top of frozen milk to keep the frozen milk from defrosting.

4) Collect 3 1/2 ounces in a 4-ounce bottle and label as to date started. Plastic bottles or double bagged nurser bags may be used.

5) Milk can be kept in refrigerator for only 24 hours.

6) Milk may be kept in the back of a freezer for 6 months.

7) To defrost milk, run under cold water, then warm water, and shake gently. When warm, give to baby.

8) Discard any defrosted breast milk the baby does not drink.

9) For transport, fresh breast milk should be carried in an insulated bag. Frozen breast milk should be packed in ice.

19. Discuss the purpose and procedure for the use of binders if the client has been instructed to use them by her physician/practitioner.
    a. Purpose: Binders are wide cloth bandages or cloth wrappings, usually of cotton, that may be worn for various purposes.
        1) Binders may be used postoperatively or after childbirth to give support to a weakened body part.
        2) They may be used to hold dressings and bandages in place.
        3) Binders may put pressure on parts of the body as a comfort measure. They could possibly be used for a nonbreastfeeding client or a client who must stop breastfeeding suddenly. Binders may also be used to keep pressure against an incision to assist with greater movement.
    b. Procedure
        1) The binder must be wrinkle-free, dry, and clean for comfort and to prevent irritated areas or bedsores.
        2) An abdominal binder is usually applied from the bottom up and may be pinned (***use caution***) or fastened with Velcro.
        3) Breast binder
            (a) A breast binder may be fastened with pins (***use caution***) or Velcro.
            (b) Fasten at the shoulders.
            (c) Work from the middle then to top and bottom.
        4) If the physician/practitioner has instructed the client to use a binder and she cannot obtain one, you may substitute a sheet, pillowcase, etc. The client must approve such items for use.
        5) Note actions in the Home Health Aide's Progress Note.

20. Discuss specific hygienic needs of the postpartum client.
    a. Vaginal delivery
        1) The client will shower according to her needs.
        2) The client will have been instructed by her physician/practitioner to wash the genital area after voiding or moving bowels.
            (a) Usually some type of squirt bottle is very useful for this.
            (b) The spray should be directed from front to back.
    b. Cesarean section delivery
    A client delivering by cesarean section should shower daily to prevent accumulation of germs on her body and around the wound that may contribute to infection.

21. Identify normal discomforts in the postpartum period and comfort measures that may be used. (See Table 3-4.)

22. Identify the procedure for application of the warm water bottle and warm compress.
    a. Method of applying warm water bottle

TABLE 3-4
Discomforts of the Postpartal Period and Relief Measures

Discomfort	Client Comfort Measure[1]	Consultation with Supervisor Required	Documentation in Progress Note Required
Episiotomy or laceration	Apply ice to painful area	yes	yes
	Assist client with her sitz bath	no	yes
Engorged breasts	Take warm shower	no	yes (no, if client takes shower to help with this)
	Apply warm compresses to upper portion of breast.	no	yes
	Hand expressing.	no	yes
	Breast massage.	no	yes
Hemmorhoids	Sit in warm tub (remember to clean feet).	no	yes
	Sit in cold or warm water sitz bath.	yes	yes
	Apply cold pack of ice chips in plastic to area.	yes	yes
Sore nipples	Use warm salt-water soaks.	yes	yes
	Change the infant's position.	no	yes
	Breaking infant suction.	no	yes
	Apply cool wet teabags to nipples.	yes	yes
	Use cream on nipples as recommended by physician/ practitioner (apply cream around nipple, not on it).	no	yes
Afterbirth pain (caused by shrinking uterus)	Apply warm compress or water bottle to abdomen.	yes	yes
	Have a massage to help relax.	no	yes
	Use pillows to aid positioning while nursing.	no	yes
Constipation	Drink 12 glasses of water a day.	no	yes
	Follow a diet that includes fresh vegetables, fruits, roughage; encourage client in limited ambulation.	yes	yes
Voiding difficulties[2]	Prepare clean warm compress (e.g., place towel on abdomen while client is on toilet).	no	yes
	Allow sink water to run while patient is on toilet.	no	yes
	Use peribottle filled with warm water while client is on toilet; spray genital area front to back.	no	yes
Exhaustion	Try to avoid disturbing client so that her needs for rest can be met adequately.	no	yes
	Offer to take care of baby while client is sleeping.	no	yes
Incisional pain	Assist client to move about in bed.	no	yes
	Offer diversional activities such as playing the radio softly, listening to music, TV, reading; talking and listening to client.	no	yes
	Massage bony prominences; place pillow between legs while client lies on her side.	no	yes
	Offer pillows to help with positioning; especially while nursing.	no	yes
	Show client how to use pillow to support incision.	no	yes
	Assist client to get into a comfortable body position.	no	yes
Itching skin due to increased bedrest	Provide clean sheets.	no	yes
	Keep bedding clean, dry, and free of crumbs.	no	yes
	Encourage and assist client in ambulation.	no	yes
	Assist client with skin hygiene.	no	yes

[1]You may suggest or assist in care.
[2]If comfort measures are unsuccessful, client should be instructed to consult with physician/practitioner; homemaker should consult agency.

1) Verify with agency before action.
2) Assemble the equipment.
   (a) Warm water bottle (may be disposable).
   (b) Pitcher of water at 102°F.
   (c) Flannel or towel cover for water bottle.
3) Wash your hands.
4) Tell the patient that you are going to apply a warm water bottle.
5) Water in the pitcher should be 102°F. Check the temperature with a bath thermometer or your elbow.
6) Fill the warm water bottle half full of water.
7) There are two methods for squeezing air out of the bottle.
   (a) Place the bag on the edge of a counter. Have the part of the bag containing the water hanging down. Place the part of the bag without the water lying on the countertop. Put your hand on top of the bag at the edge of the counter. Move your hand slowly toward the opening of the bag, pressing out the air. With the other hand, close the bag.
   (b) Place the warm water bottle in a horizontal position on a flat surface. Hold the neck of the warm water bottle upright until you can see water in the neck of the bottle. (The water squeezes out the air.)
8) Fasten the top tightly.
9) Dry the warm water bottle. Check for leaks by turning it upside down.
10) Place the warm water bottle in the flannel cover or wrap it in the towel.
11) Apply it gently to the proper body area.
12) Never place the warm water bottle on top of a painful area. The weight will increase the pain. Place it on the side.
13) Check the skin in 10 to 15 minutes to be sure temperature is correct and there is no evidence of burning.
14) Check the warm water bottle every hour to be sure the temperature is correct. Change the water in the bottle when necessary to continue treatment at the same temperature.
15) Check the skin under the warm water bottle every hour. If the skin is red, remove the water bottle and report to your Healthcare Supervisor.
16) Clean standard equipment and put it in its proper place. Discard disposable equipment.
17) Make the patient comfortable.
18) Wash your hands.
19) Document treatment on the Homemaker's Progress Note.
   (a) Time the warm water bottle was applied
   (b) Length of treatment
   (c) Area of application

20) Remove the bottle if the skin appears too red or the client complains of bottle being "too warm."

21) Report to your Home Care Supervisor observations of anything unusual.

b. Method of applying wet warm compress

1) Follow the general procedures for applying a warm water bottle, but equipment will include the following items instead of those for a warm water bottle.

(a) Towel-type material large enough to cover the area (peripads may be used for small areas)

(b) Some kind of clean plastic to place over the compress for heat retention

2) Dip the towel material into tested warm water and wring out well.

3) Cover the area with the warm towel and completely cover the compress with plastic.

4) Check the skin after 10 to 15 minutes for temperature.

5) Remove the compress if the skin appears too red or the client complains it is "too warm."

23. Identify procedures for application of cold as a comfort measure.

a. Dry cold: Ice bag with ice chips or a solution frozen in a container

1) Wash your hands.

2) Rinse ice bag or container and check for leaks. Fill ice bag with chips or fill a container with water and freeze.

3) Fill bag or container only half full. Force out the remaining air. Secure the top.

4) Always cover bag or container with a towel, then apply. Check frequently. If the treated area becomes white or blue, immediately remove the dry cold application.

b. Wet cold: Cold compresses
Follow the directions for a wet warm compress except in regard to solution temperature. Mix the cold compress solution and add ice chips. Keep it cold. Don't let the solution become too diluted. Add more solution as necessary.

24. Identify postpartum problems that require investigation by the physician/practitioner.

a. Vaginal bleeding soaking more than one pad per hour should be reported.

b. A foul or unusual odor to lochia (vaginal bleeding) is also important to report to the physician/practitioner.

c. The inability to void or completely empty bladder needs investigation as well.

d. A flulike feeling, fever, or chills should be referred to the physician/practitioner.

e. A fever above 100.4°F for more than a day requires attention. (Fever up to 100.4°F may occur for a day when the milk comes in.)

f. Any redness/tenderness of the breast or a reddened lump in the breast should be reported.

g. Any change in the odor and/or color in breast milk needs investigation.

h. Extreme tenderness of the episiotomy also requires the physician/practitioner's attention.

i. Tenderness above the pubic bone, accompanied by frequency and/or urgency when urinating should be referred to the physician/practitioner.

j. If any part of the incision becomes separated, call the physician/practitioner.

k. Drainage from the surgical incision requires medical attention.

l. Increased redness or warmness of the incision should be reported.

25. Discuss the emotional needs of the postpartum woman.

a. Rest is necessary, because sleep deprivation decreases the ability to cope with responsibilities.

b. Positive reinforcement will support the client in feeling that she is doing things the "right" way.

c. Knowing that her family is being taken care of will help set the client's mind at ease.

d. Time with the other children will help the client.

e. Entertainment (TV, books, etc.) will relax the postpartum woman.

f. Time for parent/infant bonding is very important.

g. Having someone to "listen" is another need of the postpartum woman.

26. Discuss the procedure for giving a bed bath.
If a client is unable to take a shower or tub bath, she may request a bed bath. Let the patient bathe herself as much as possible. Bathing is good exercise for a patient confined to bed. It also gives you a chance to observe the client's condition and increases the client's circulation. In some cases, you will have to assist the client or bathe her completely. Follow these guidelines.

a. Place on the bedside table all of the necessary items: a washbasin with warm water, a washcloth, soap, towels, a cotton blanket, skin lotion, clean pajamas or clothing, and toilet articles. If the patient has a dry skin problem, baby oil may be added to the bath water. Be sure the room is warm.

b. Talk to the client and put her at ease while bathing. Maintain modesty at all times.

c. Place a towel under the client's head and neck. Wash her face, neck, and ears. Rinse and dry completely. Make a mitt with the washcloth so as not to have flapping ends dripping on the client.

d. Remove the bedcovers and the client's pajamas. Cover the client with the cotton blanket. Uncover each part of the body only when it is to be washed. Place a towel under the portion of the client's body you will wash next. Wash and rinse and dry completely. Apply lotion to dry skin areas, such as feet, elbows, and heels. Cover her with a cotton blanket.

e. Wash the client's body in this sequence: hands and arms, chest, abdomen, feet. Change the water and turn the client. Wash her back and buttocks. Have the client wash the genitals. Give gentle back care, showing special attention to reddened areas, especially the buttocks. Turn the client and put on her pajamas or clothing.

f. Cover the client with the sheet and blanket. Assist the client with her personal toileting, such as combing her hair. Wash your hands.

g. When bathing a client, remember these points.

1) Clean the areas in creases and fat folds such as under the breasts and between fingers and toes.

2) Notice the condition of the skin. If a bony area is reddened, rub it frequently with a lotion.

3) Never rub the client's legs. Postpartum women can be prone to phlebitis. Rubbing may cause clots to be freed into the bloodstream and enter the lungs (pulmonary emboli), heart (heart attack), or brain (stroke). Check to determine that the OB care provider is aware of any reddened, warm areas on the legs.
4) Support the client's limbs under the joints during the bath.
5) Keep all nails cleaned and filed. Nails may be trimmed with permission of the nurse in charge.
6) Change the water often. Don't let it get cold or soapy. Soapy rinse water dries out the skin and causes irritation.
6) Record and report to your Home Care Supervisor any skin changes.

CHAPTER 4

Home Health Aide–Family Teaching Materials

The teaching materials found in this chapter are meant to be copied and distributed to Home Health Aides and the families they assist. These are only a few of the teaching tools one can access with a little research. Excellent materials can be found through The Division of Maternal Child Health, Health and Human Services (5600 Fishers Lane, Rockville, Maryland 20857). In addition, further resources should be available through state and local health departments. Visual and written aids assist the Home Health Aide in the educational process by stimulating multiple senses and thus increasing stimulation of the memory.

Keep in mind that these items are simply *tools*. They are meant to assist in the educational process, in both the Home Health Aide training program and with the client. Do not assume the client can read or has developed an adequate trusting relationship with you to value your information. Persons providing home care work in the domain of the client, not the office or the hospital. The Home Health Aide's ability to communicate and develop the "helping relationship" is crucial to success in providing care.

PARENT EDUCATION PROGRAM: PRETERM LABOR

What Is Preterm Labor and What Does It Mean to My Baby?

Once your OB care provider has diagnosed preterm labor, you probably have many questions. This information is provided to help you understand the diagnosis of preterm labor as well as to help you identify more questions that you might want to ask your OB care provider or nurse. The information here is also designed to help you understand and deal with the treatment plan you might need to follow.

What Does Preterm Mean?

Pregnancy is calculated to be 40 weeks from the first day of your last period. Any delivery beyond the 37th week is considered term. Any delivery that occurs during the period of 20 to 36 weeks is considered preterm. Preterm birth is one of the most important problems affecting newborns today. Some of the complications include respiratory difficulties, feeding problems, infections, and problems with temperature regulation. This is why it is so important to provide this information for you, so that you can have the tools to help identify, treat, and prevent preterm labor and birth.

Am I at Risk?

The cause of preterm labor and birth is not exactly understood, but certain situations have been identified as increasing your risk for preterm labor. The following have been associated with an increased risk of preterm labor.

1. A previous preterm labor or delivery
2. An abnormally shaped uterus, DES daughters (daughters of women who took the drug diethylstilbestrol while they were pregnant), uterine surgery
3. Two or more second trimester abortions or miscarriages
4. Incompetent cervix, cone biopsy, large fibroids
5. Current pregnancy with twins, triplets, etc.
6. The feeling that something is wrong even without any specific symptoms or cause

How Can I Check for Contractions?

Lie down and place your fingers on your uterus. If your uterus is tightening and softening you will be able to tell how often it is happening. Time the contractions by noting the time between the start of one tightening and the start of the next tightening. Because at times uterine contractions (especially in preterm labor) occur without any other warning sign, it is important that you feel your abdomen for contractions (or use home monitoring if that is part of your treatment) at least twice a day for half-hour periods. It is very helpful to do this at the same time each day if possible.

How Will I Be Treated If I Have Preterm Labor?

Sometimes preterm labor may be treated with rest and modification of your activities. You might need to increase your rest time. Rest on your side at least twice a day in the morning and afternoon. You might need to modify or stop work or school activities. You will need to discuss with your OB care provider or nurse how long your rest periods need to be. Many times bedrest at home is recommended. That can be more difficult than you could imagine. You will need to adjust many aspects of your life. The temporary reorganization of your activities might need to include stopping work, managing your household from bed, physical reorganization of your house, and assistance with the care of your children. An excellent book available to you that contains lots of practical ideas and answers to many questions is *Pregnancy Bedrest,* a guide for the pregnant woman and her family written by Susan H. Johnston and Deborah A. Kraut. This book is available at your local bookstore.

Will I Have to Be Admitted to the Hospital?

Sometimes you might need to be hospitalized and treated with medications for your preterm labor. Medications that will be used are called tocolytics (brethine, terbutaline, ritodrine, yutopar, or magnesium sulfate). These medications stop labor by relaxing the muscles of the uterus. Like many medications, they will affect your body with additional side effects.

1. You may experience a faster heartbeat, tremors, nausea, vomiting, headache, and flushing of the skin.
2. You might experience other symptoms such as nervousness, jitteriness, restlessness, anxiety, tiredness, listlessness, stomach discomforts, difficulty in breathing, drowsiness, and weakness, but these are less common.

It is very important that you discuss the medications with your OB care provider or nurse so that you know exactly what you are taking, how often you should take your medication, and what to expect with the particular medication you are taking. It is possible to receive tocolytic medication via a small pump that delivers the medication under your skin. The use of this pump allows for very small amounts of medication to be delivered more frequently.

The feelings you might experience can range anywhere from fear and tremendous guilt to anger and frustration. Many women report feeling numb and helpless as the diagnosis is first presented to them. Many ask, "Why me?" "What have I done to go through this?" Your expectations and hopes for your unborn child can often change into incredible fear for the health of your baby. You will probably always feel a sense of threat to the pregnancy and often wonder if you will be a mother of a healthy baby. You might at times also feel inadequate because you might not be able to maintain a safe environment for your baby. All of these feelings are normal and are very common in women experiencing preterm labor or high-risk pregnancy. The feelings of loss of the "perfect pregnancy" are experienced by many women; many women also feel guilt because they think they have somehow caused preterm labor. It is important that you understand that these feelings are normal in your situation and that you are not the only person who has ever felt this way before. It might be helpful for you to discuss your feelings with your OB care provider or nurse.

The father of the new baby may experience the same fears and concerns for you and the baby. He is often asked to be the main source of emotional support for you and your family. Many fathers feel jealous and guilty at the same time. The feelings of jealousy of the baby and your preoccupation with the pregnancy are many times accompanied by a feeling of guilt over these feelings. Fathers often will feel protective of their partners and at the same time anxious about whether they will be able to provide the care that mother and baby might need.

The effect of your hospitalization on your family can be tremendous. Family members might feel left out in the high-tech care environment of the hospital. It is important that you enlist their care and support, as much as they are able to provide for you. It is also very important that you attempt to spend as much time as possible with your children to help them maintain their feeling of importance to the family. Discussion of all your feelings between you and your partner as well as with the family is very important to the protection of your family unit.

PARENT EDUCATION PROGRAM: KEGEL EXERCISES

The primary muscle involved in Kegel exercises is the pubococcygeus (P-C) muscle. Exercising the P-C muscle provides the following benefits.

1. Urinary sphincter control is strengthened.
2. Muscle tone in the vagina is increased.
3. The ability to constrict the vagina voluntarily is also increased. This increases female vaginal perception and response during penile–vaginal intercourse.
4. Exercising the P-C muscle contributes to the elimination of pain during sexual intercourse.
5. Exercising the P-C muscle increases the ability to relax the pelvic floor, which aids in the birth of the baby.
6. Kegel exercises also speed up the postpartum recovery of pelvic floor muscle tone.

To identify the P-C muscle, sit on the toilet with your legs spread as far apart as possible. Start and stop the flow of urine. The P-C muscle is the only one that can accomplish this while in this position. Contract the P-C muscle, hold for 3 seconds, relax, and repeat this process. Because the P-C is a muscle like other muscles, with overly strenuous exercise it can become sore. If this happens, either stop doing the exercise for 1 or 2 days until the temporary soreness disappears and then resume, or reduce substantially the number of exercises done per day and then gradually increase to the recommended number.

Once you learn where the P-C muscle is, Kegel exercises can be done during daily activities that do not involve a great deal of moving around (e.g., driving an automobile, sitting, doing dishes, watching TV, waiting in a checkout line, lying in bed). Practice the Kegel exercises five times a day (15 contractions each time) or 10 contractions each time you open the refrigerator. Soon Kegels will become second nature to you.

PARENT EDUCATION PROGRAM: POSTPARTUM INSTRUCTIONS FOR MOTHERS

Rest

1. The new mother should get plenty of rest for the first couple of weeks.
2. The client should care for herself and her baby only; she shouldn't expect too much of herself.
3. The new mother should obtain help for general household duties (cleaning, cooking, laundry, shopping, and caring for older children).
4. Emphasize that the new mother needs to rest when the baby is sleeping.
5. Limit visitors to relatives and close friends.
6. Remember, fatigue decreases the milk supply and the ability to cope with new and added responsibilities.

Activity

1. Limit stair climbing for the first week.
2. The client should let her body be the guide for activity and exercise.
3. The new mother may go out to dinner or for a ride but she should not drive for 1 to 2 weeks unless otherwise instructed by her physician. Cesarean section patients should verify with their OB care provider when driving is permitted.

Diet

1. Advise the client to drink 8 to 10 glasses of water per day.
2. Her diet should consist of protein, fruits, vegetables, and milk.
3. A small bowl of bran daily will prevent constipation
4. The client should continue taking prenatal vitamins daily at least until the postpartum exam. If the OB care provider has not instructed her to do so, the client should verify this with her physician.
5. An adequate diet as shown above is important, particularly if the mother is breastfeeding, because it takes about 800 calories daily to produce the milk the baby needs.
6. Remember, if the new mother does not eat, she will become fatigued and milk volume will decrease.

Vaginal Discharge

1. At first discharge is red, like a heavy period, for 1 to 3 days.

2. By the 3rd day the discharge should have thinned and lightened in color.

3. By the 10th day the discharge is often a pale pink, watery fluid, heavy enough to wear a light pad.

4. If, after the 3rd day, bleeding becomes bright red and heavy again, it is often a sign that the new mother has done too much and should slow down and rest.

Intercourse

1. For the majority of women, intercourse may be resumed when the vaginal area feels comfortable and the episiotomy has healed. She should check any doubts with her physician.

2. Gentleness and added lubrication may be needed for comfort when sexual activity is first resumed.

3. Breastfeeding mothers may ovulate before their first menstrual period, therefore it is possible to get pregnant again even before menstruation has resumed.

4. Foam and condoms will provide contraception if sexual activity is resumed before 6 weeks postpartum.

5. Birth control can be discussed at the 6-week postpartum visit.

Baths and Showers

1. The new mother may shower as necessary, but stress two points. ***Do not*** take a tub bath for at least 3 days unless otherwise instructed by the OB care provider. ***Do not*** use bubble bath or oils in the bath water.

2. Warm showers may help to relieve the discomfort of breast engorgement.

3. ***Do not use douches!!!***

Stitches and Hemorrhoids

1. Warm tub baths or sitz baths are recommended several times a day.

2. For discomfort of hemorrhoids use Nupercainol cream, Dermoplast, or Tucks pads. The client should consult her OB care provider.

3. There is no cause for alarm if a week or two postpartum loose stitches are found on a pad or in the toilet.

4. Reassure the new mother that stitches normally are absorbed or loosen when they no longer are needed.

Postpartum Blues

1. The new mother may experience postpartum blues during the first 10 days postpartum. The most common symptom is unexpected and unexplainable crying. Also, she may feel irritable.

2. Postpartum blues usually go away about 72 hours after onset, but they may continue for as long as 10 days.

3. If postpartum blues symptoms persist or increase in severity, they may be an early sign of postpartum depression.

4. Postpartum depression is experienced by 10% of all women and may occur anywhere within 6 months after delivery.

5. Signs and symptoms of postpartum depression
   a. Sleep disturbances may occur.
   b. Loss of appetite is common.
   c. Fear and anxiety are also signs of postpartum depression.
   d. A feeling of hopelessness may develop.
   e. Hostility or self-blame are also common.
   f. Difficulty concentrating or making decisions is another sign.

6. The client may want to seek professional help if the signs and symptoms of postpartum depression are experienced.

Baby's Fussy Periods

1. The baby may go through fussy periods during the day or evening.

2. Fussy periods may happen because the mother's milk supply is low at the end of the day.

3. The new mother may need to nurse more frequently.

4. Use calming tactics such as rocking, walking, strollers, swings, etc.

5. Lay the baby down to see if he or she will sleep.

   "Recent research shows that SIDS is more common in babies who go to sleep on their tummies. By making sure your baby goes to sleep on its back or side, you can help reduce the risk of SIDS." (*Back to Sleep: Reducting the Risk of Sudden Infant Death Syndrome—What You Can Do.* U.S. Public Health Service, the American Academy of Pediatrics, the SIDS Alliance, and the Association of SIDS Program Professionals.). If you have any questions about your baby's sleep position, contact your health care provider first. Then you can call toll free 1-800-505-CRIB, or write to Back to Sleep, P.O Box 29111, Washington D.C. 20040, for more information.

Postpartum Problems

Call your healthcare provider if any of the following problems occur.

1. A flulike feeling, fever, or chills

2. A foul-smelling discharge or unusual abdominal tenderness

3. Redness and tenderness of the breasts
4. Extreme tenderness of the episiotomy area
5. Tenderness of the pubic bone, accompanied by frequency, urgency, and burning with urination

These symptoms may indicate an infection of some type, which requires professional attention and treatment.

PARENT EDUCATION PROGRAM: NEWBORN INSTRUCTIONS

Bathing

1. Sponge bathe the newborn with mild soap (low alkaline) such as Dove or Castille until the cord has fallen off and the area is completely healed.
2. Do not use oil or powder on the baby's head or skin.
3. When the navel is healed, the baby may have a tub bath.
4. Bathe the baby before feeding.

Cord Care

1. The cord usually falls off within 7 to 10 days.
2. Use alcohol and cotton to cleanse and bathe the area around the base of the cord at every diaper change.
3. There may be one or two drops of blood when the cord separates.
4. Keep the diaper folded beneath the navel to facilitate drying of the cord.
5. Call the pediatric care provider if the cord has a foul odor or if the skin of the abdominal area around the umbilical cord becomes red.

Diaper Rash

1. Change the baby's diaper when it is soiled.
2. Avoid using plastic pants when possible or change the baby frequently. Air the buttocks when changing.
3. Diapers should be washed with mild soap and rinsed well after each laundering.
4. Apply Balmex or Desitin to the diaper area, especially the creases, at each diaper change (Vaseline can be used all the time on the diaper area).

Circumcision

Apply Vaseline liberally at every diaper change until the area is no longer red or swollen.

Nails

1. Use an emery board to file nails. They are too soft to cut with scissors for the first couple of weeks.
2. Never cut with cuticle scissors

Clothing

1. Keep the baby warm, but do not overheat.
2. Use simple, easily washed clothes.
3. On hot days, a diaper and T-shirt may be enough.
4. The baby should wear one more layer of clothing than his or her mother.
5. If it is cool and breezy, the baby's head should be covered.

Feeding

1. If breastfeeding, refer to instructions and information on breastfeeding.
2. Hold the baby at every feeding.
3. Feed the baby when he or she is hungry (usually every 3 to 5 hours).
4. Do not wake the baby at night.
5. Burp the baby after every $^1/_2$ to 1 ounce at first.
6. Place the baby on his or her stomach or right side (roll the blanket and place behind the back for support).
7. Do not start any new foods (cereal, juice, or fruit) until the pediatric care provider gives permission.
8. Use formula as ordered by the pediatric care provider. The powdered form may be more economical. The client should always follow the instructions on the can for mixing and preparing the formula.
9. The baby may have 1 to 2 ounces of boiled, cooled water if fussy.

Bowel Movements

1. The breastfed baby's bowel movements are normally loose and unformed.
2. The breastfed baby may have several small movements each day or may go for several days without having a bowel movement at all.
3. A totally breastfed baby is never constipated and seldom has diarrhea (watery bowel movements). Relax with your infant. He or she will adjust to you. If you are tense, the baby will feel tense; if you are relaxed, it will help relax your baby.

PARENT EDUCATION PROGRAM: BREASTFEEDING

Position for Breastfeeding

1. Assume a comfortable position (sitting, lying, football hold); positions should be rotated to avoid stress or sore nipples.

2. Bring the baby to the nipple. You may want to use pillows. This avoids the stress of the baby pulling on the nipples.

3. Expose the breast. Support the baby's head in the crook of the arm, with the other hand supporting the nipple in a scissorslike hold or thumb and forefinger hold.

4. Compress the breast if it is large, with the finger at the baby's nose to prevent obstruction of breathing.

5. Timing
   a. Feed for 5 minutes per side on the first day.
   b. Feed for 7 to 8 minutes per side on the second day.
   c. Feed for 10 minutes per side on the third day.
   d. Build up to 20 minutes per side.
   e. If the baby falls asleep at 10 minutes, when milk comes in cut back to 5 minutes per side.
   f. If the baby is still hungry, you may go back to the first side for another 5 minutes.
   g. Nurse both breasts at each feeding. Start with the breast you ended with at the last feeding.
   h. At end of the feeding, break the suction by placing your finger in the corner of the baby's mouth.
   i. Air dry the nipples after each feeding and apply Eucerin cream around the areola (brown area) but not on the tip of the nipple. This will keep the nipples from becoming tender.

Breast Massage and Hand Expression

1. Breast massage must be used to bring the milk down to the baby, to relieve fullness, and before pumping or hand expressing to decrease the time spent on collection.

2. To massage: Place one hand under the breast. With the other hand, stroke down toward the nipple, starting from the shoulder. Then stroke under the breast and up. Do this for 1 minute.

3. To hand express: Put the thumb and forefinger on the areola about 1 inch from the nipple. Press back toward the chest wall and squeeze together to compress the milk sinus.

Milk Collection and Storage

1. Milk may be collected and stored when mothers work or are not going to be home for feedings and want the baby to drink from a bottle.
2. Collect milk by hand expression, breast pump, or with milk cups. One ounce at a time may be accumulated, so make sure that enough time is allotted.
3. Collect in a clean container.
4. Chill milk, then freeze. Chilled milk may be poured on top of frozen.
5. Milk may be stored in the refrigerator for 24 to 48 hours only.
6. Glass or plastic bottles or double bagged nursers may be used.
7. Milk can be kept in the back of the freezer for several months.
8. To defrost, run under cold, then warm water, then shake.
9. Discard defrosted milk that the baby does not use.
10. Milk to be transported should be placed in an insulated bag, frozen, or packed with ice.

Breastfeeding Solutions and Problems

1. Soreness
   a. Nipples may become red and cracked or bleeding. The nipple may be sore until it becomes accustomed to baby's sucking, or soreness may be due to poor positioning, removing the baby from the breast improperly, not allowing the nipples to dry, or irritants such as soap, shampoo, rough clothing, plastic liners in bras, or harsh laundry detergents.
   b. Solutions
      1) Rotate the position of the baby when feeding.
      2) Provide short, frequent feedings.
      3) Make sure the baby has the large portion of the nipple in the mouth, not just the tip.
      4) Make sure the baby's mouth is close to the nipple to avoid pulling on the nipple.
      5) Air dry the nipples and use Eucerin cream as necessary.
      6) Nurse on the least sore side first.
      7) Always break suction before removing the baby.
      8) Try saline soaks, ice on the nipples before feeding, a nipple shield or Vitamin E oil if the nipple becomes cracked or bleeds.
2. Fullness or engorgement
   a. Breasts become full on the second or third day postpartum, when the milk comes in. Engorgement is when the milk becomes backed up and the breast and nipples become hard and shiny.
   b. Solutions
      1) Short, frequent feedings help. Do not miss feedings, and nurse on both sides each feeding.

2) Warm showers, compresses, massage, and expression relieve the fullness.
3) Make sure the bra is not cutting or binding in any place.
4) Occasionally expressing or pumping after feeding may relieve fullness.

3. Plugged duct
   a. A plugged duct produces a lump or tenderness in one spot.
   b. Solution
      1) Nurse on the affected breast first.
      2) Direct the baby's chin toward the lump when nursing.
      3) Avoid tight bras, underwire bras, and bunching clothing.
      4) Use massage and heat while nursing to encourage lump drain.

4. Breast infection
   a. Symptoms: flulike feeling, redness, tenderness and fever. The condition may be aggravated by not emptying the breast completely, abrupt weaning, or the mother's fatigue.
   b. Solutions
      1) Heat: warm, moist compresses may help.
      2) Rest will alleviate the mother's fatigue, helping her condition.
      3) Empty the breast completely; when nursing, direct the baby's chin toward a sore spot or lump.
      4) If the client's temperature increases to 100°, call the physician.

Growth Spurts

1. Growth spurts usually come within the first 10 days, at 3 weeks, at 3 months, and at 6 months.
2. The baby may want to nurse more often.
3. Nurse the baby on demand to build up the milk supply.
4. Do not give supplemental feeding, because this may interfere with establishment of an adequate milk supply. The more frequently the breasts are emptied, the more milk is produced.

PARENT EDUCATION PROGRAM: EXPRESSING BREAST MILK

Breast milk may be expressed and collected for later use by hand expression, a hand-operated breast pump, or a semi-automatic battery-operated or electric breast pump. A sterile container, such as sterile plastic bottle bags (Playtex or Gerber liners) or a sterilized plastic or glass bottle, should be used to collect the milk. Before collecting milk, wash your hands with soap and water and dry them thoroughly.

Massage each breast in this way. If large-breasted, support the breast with one hand. Beginning at the chest wall, use the other flattened hand to exert gentle pressure on the breast toward the nipple, working around the breast. Work in the areas of greatest milk duct development, under the breast and along the side under the arm. Use the palms of the hands, not the fingers, for firm pressure. (These instructions come from *Counseling the Nursing Mother*, Lauwers and Woessner, 1983, p. 411.)

Stimulate the let-down reflex or milk ejection reflex by gently rolling and tugging the nipples between your thumb and forefinger. Dripping of milk from the nipples is one sign that the let-down or milk ejection reflex is working. When you feel that the let-down reflex has begun to work, you can begin expressing breast milk by the chosen method.

Collecting milk may take about 20 minutes. Alternate the breast from which you are expressing milk about four times; when the milk flow slows down on one breast, switch to the other breast.

A breast pump collection kit should be washed daily in soap and water and rinsed between uses. A dishwasher (which leaves no soap residue) provides an excellent method for cleaning the kit. When collecting milk for a hospitalized infant, the collection kit must the sterilized daily.

PARENT EDUCATION PROGRAM: STORAGE OF HUMAN MILK

Containers

For hospitalized infants, ask your baby's nurse for storage containers. For home use, the following containers and methods are recommended.

1. Clean heavy plastic or glass containers.
2. Disposable bottle liners; double bags are more sturdy.
3. Seal with a lid or twist tie and store upright until frozen.
4. Label the container with the date on which the milk was expressed

Storage

For hospitalized infants, milk should be refrigerated within 1 hour of expressing. In general, use the following guidelines.

1. Milk may be kept at room temperature.
   a. Colostrum: 12 to 24 hours
   b. Mature milk: 6 to 10 hours
2. Milk may be refrigerated.
   a. Home use: up to 5 days
   b. Hospitalized infants: up to 48 hours
3. Milk may be frozen.
   a. Home use: 2 weeks in a freezer compartment located inside a refrigerator
   b. Home use: 6 months in a refrigerator/freezer with separate doors (frost free)
   c. Home use: 6 months to 1 year in a deep freeze, 0°F or below
   d. Hospitalized infants: 3 months

Warming Milk

Thaw and/or heat milk by placing the container in warm water. Human milk heats to a comfortable feeding temperature in about 10 minutes.

HOME VISITS PROTOCOL: EDUCATING PARENTS AND/OR CAREGIVERS ABOUT DIARRHEA AND NUTRITION

The major complication from gastroenteritis is dehydration and accompanying electrolyte imbalance. Signs of dehydration may not always be apparent to parents. Parents should be informed of these signs and should report them. Assessment data provide the basis for decision making pertaining to treatment and care concerning infant diarrhea and nutrition. One-to-one teaching that is culturally sensitive and that uses language the caregiver can easily understand is the goal.

Criteria

Home visits are recommended in cases of infants presenting to the emergency room with the following conditions.

1. Acute gastroenteritis (AGE)
2. Vomiting (with no evidence of intestinal obstruction or acute abdomen)
3. Poor intake
4. Dehydration (excluding those patients exhibiting signs of circulatory collapse)

Recommended Visit Pattern

Daily visits are suggested to monitor intake, output, and daily weight; to provide physical assessments; and to ensure compliance with the treatment regime.

PARENT EDUCATION PROGRAM: DIARRHEA

Diarrhea is one of the most common problems in infants, as well as one of the most potentially dangerous. The following information should be helpful in understanding exactly what is going on in the child's body, how to treat diarrhea, and how not to treat diarrhea.

Diarrhea and Dehydration

1. Definition of diarrhea: Three or more liquid stools (liquid bowel movements) in a day.
2. Causes of diarrhea
   a. Germs, bacterial or viral, that cause an infection of the intestines (bowels). This is called gastroenteritis.
   b. Microscopic animal organisms. Giardia is a common cause of a highly contagious diarrhea often transmitted from infant to infant in day care centers.
   c. Fungus (candida is one species) can cause diarrhea, especially in infants who have been weakened by other illnesses or who have immune-deficiency diseases.

d. Parasitic worms are very common among infants, who tend to put their unwashed fingers and hands in or near their mouths.

e. Physiologic causes include fever. Many infants get diarrhea along with a cold, change in diet, milk intolerance, or rich or spicy foods.

Regardless of the cause, diarrhea should stop within a week. If it continues, call the infant's doctor or clinic.

3. Impact of diarrhea on the infant's health

   a. Colds and diarrhea are the two most common illnesses of infants. Worldwide, infants have 1 to 10 episodes of diarrhea a year.

   b. Diarrhea can cause dehydration from fluid loss.

   c. Common diarrhea can cause serious illness or even death, especially in very young infants. In the United States, 200,000 infants per year are hospitalized and 500 infants die as a result of dehydration from diarrhea. This can be prevented if pediatric care providers and caregivers understand diarrhea, dehydration, and simple steps they can take to prevent them.

4. Definition/explanation of dehydration

   a. At birth, the human body is about 80% water. By 9 months, it is 60% water and should stay at that level.

   b. Electrolytes are special kinds of salts (sodium and potassium) in the body that are vital to the body's systems.

   c. Diarrhea causes body fluids and electrolytes to be lost in the stool. This can cause dehydration and even death.

5. Signs of dehydration (indicating a lack of fluid)

   a. Dry mouth (lips or tongue)

   b. Unusual drowsiness, listlessness, or fussiness

   c. Extreme thirst

   d. Sunken-looking eyes

   e. Decreased urination (or less than six wet diapers per day or a period of longer than 4 hours without urination)

   f. Concentrated urine (urine is very dark yellow)

   g. Absence of tears

   h. Rapid heartbeat or pulse

   i. Sunken soft spot (fontanel)

   j. Poor skin turgor (pinch skin on abdomen; the skin should return to normal after being released)

6. What to do if an infant is dehydrated.

   a. If an infant with diarrhea appears dehydrated, has a fever over 101°, cannot drink fluids, or has blood in the stool, call a doctor or clinic ***immediately***. Blood in the stool can make it look red, rust-colored, or flecked with blood.

   b. ***If an infant with diarrhea is unconscious, "floppy," or has a high fever (more than 103°), take the infant immediately to the nearest hospital!***

7. Management of gastroenteritis involves three components.
   a. Maintain or restore fluid and electrolyte balance.
   b. Restore the bowel to normal functioning.
   c. Prevent the infection of others in contact with the infant.

8. Care of an infant with diarrhea

   These guidelines will help you to help your infant get well, keep him or her out of the hospital, and avoid a painful needle stick for intravenous treatment.

   a. Rehydration
      To prevent and treat dehydration, start oral rehydration therapy (ORT) as soon as the diarrhea begins. ORT is discussed and explained in detail in the next section.
   b. Feeding
      1) Sometimes people think that it is necessary to "rest the gut" in cases of diarrhea. ***This is not a good practice!*** It is very important that infants eat when they are sick, even when they have diarrhea. Eating the right foods actually helps the infant get well faster. The right foods give the infant the energy needed for healing and for fighting the infection causing the diarrhea. Small, frequent feedings are most often given, yet larger quantities offered less frequently may be recommended because frequent feedings have the potential to induce peristalsis.
      2) ***DO continue to breastfeed or bottlefeed your baby normally*** (unless instructed otherwise by your baby's pediatric care provider).
      3) ***DO NOT give the infant sugary or salty foods or drinks.*** These can make the diarrhea worse.

9. Medication for diarrhea
   Diarrhea is a reaction of the intestines to an infection or irritation. The very best care for most cases of infant diarrhea is simply replacing the fluids and salts lost by giving oral rehydration solution and feeding the infant good foods while he or she is sick or following an illness.

   Parents are usually very concerned about the frequency and appearance of bowel movements and want to give the infant something to "bind" the bowels. This does not really help because, when the infant has diarrhea, the body fluid and salts are still being lost. They are just being held in the intestine longer. The fluid in the intestine does not go back into the body where it is needed! It is possible that the infant is still becoming dehydrated, even though the diarrheal bowel movements are not being expelled. So, "binding" the infant will give parents a false sense of security because it appears that the diarrhea is getting better. It is not—it is just being held inside longer. Also, you might not realize how much fluid is being lost because it is "hidden" in the intestine, so you will not realize how much the infant needs to drink.

   Remember, the main goal is to prevent dehydration and to recognize it early if it does develop.

10. Record keeping
    If your infant has diarrhea it may be helpful to keep a written record, so that if you have to call the pediatric care provider you will be prepared to ask and answer questions. Start the notes as soon as the diarrhea starts. You should record the following information.

   a. Amount and color of the stool and time
   b. Amount and kind of fluid the infant takes and time
   c. Temperature
   d. Weight
      If you have a scale, weigh the infant as soon as the diarrhea starts, especially if the infant is under 3 years old. If you have this information when you need to call the doctor, nurse, or clinic, they will be able to decide more easily if the infant should be brought in.

11. Comfort the infant
    Infants with diarrhea do not feel well and therefore have special needs. Babies' bottoms hurt and they may be cranky. These are some things you can do to prevent and treat diaper rash to make the baby feel better.
    a. Do not use baby wipes that contain alcohol.
    b. Do change diapers often.
    c. Do wash the infant's bottom with soap, rinse with plain warm water, and gently pat dry.
    d. Do apply Vaseline, Desitin, or A&D ointment to the infant's bottom. This will keep the stool away from the skin.
    e. Do apply cornstarch or baby powder to the infant's bottom.

12. Prevention of diarrhea
    The microorganisms (germs) that cause diarrhea are passed by people, objects, and food. To prevent the spread of diarrhea, here are some things you can do.
    a. Wash your hands well with soap and water.
       1) Before cooking food or feeding your infant
       2) After changing your infant's diaper or going to the toilet
       3) After handling raw meat of any kind
       4) After giving a sick infant medication or feeding
    b. Do not let infants play with, or put into their mouths, things that you know are dirty.
    c. Throw disposable diapers out immediately and keep them in a trash can away from infants and pets. The trash can should have a lid.
    d. Keep dirty cloth diapers away from infants and pets and wash them as soon as possible.
    e. Be careful how you store and prepare foods. To prevent the spread of diarrhea from food, be sure to cook and prepare foods correctly and wash dishes and utensils well after use. Foods to be especially careful with are eggs, fish and shellfish, chicken, and pork. Promptly refrigerate foods that can spoil.

Oral Rehydration Therapy (ORT)

1. Definition: Oral rehydration therapy involves drinking a special solution to replace, in the proper proportions, essential body fluids and salts lost during diarrhea to treat and ***prevent dehydration***.

2. Why ORT works: The special salts (electrolytes) and water that are lost in diarrhea are needed by the body to function properly. Drinking a balanced solution of salt, water, and sugar can prevent as well as treat dehydration of people with diarrhea. These solutions are called oral rehydration solutions (ORS) or oral electrolyte solutions (OES).

3. For the solution to work best, proper amounts of the ingredients are critical. Too little or too much of any of the ingredients will cause the solution to not work correctly. (This is why an infant with diarrhea should not have salty or sugary foods and drinks and why plain water is not enough.) However, fluids are critical, and oral rehydration solution is the best replacement fluid. If ORS is not available, then any fluid is better than none.

4. Oral rehydration solutions
   a. What they are
      1) Oral rehydration solutions are special mixtures of water and electrolytes in the correct quantities that will replace the fluids and salts lost in diarrhea.
      2) Commercial brands of ORS are available, including Pedialyte, Ricelyte, and generic brands, which can be found in grocery stores and drug stores.
      3) ***There is also a solution that you can make at home*** that is a good substitute for commercial brands when it is made according to the directions. It is very ***easy*** and ***inexpensive*** to make; the recipe is provided below.
   b. How and when to give them to infants
      1) ***How*** you give the solution is as important as what you give to an infant. To prevent dehydration it is necessary to replace the fluid and salts lost in the stool, so it is important to give enough solution.
      2) When an infant has diarrhea, he or she may have an upset stomach. It is very important to give the solution slowly enough that it can be absorbed by the body and not cause the infant to vomit. Here is a general guide to giving an oral rehydration solution.
         (a) Encourage the infant to take the solution after each stool or every few minutes.
         (b) The solution should be taken in small amounts, either in sips or by spoon, so that it is easily absorbed. Do not let the infant gulp it down.
         (c) An infant under 24 months may need 1/4 to 1/2 cup. A child 2 to 10 years old may need 1/2 to 1 cup.
      3) Remember, the solution is replacing what is lost in the diarrhea, so if there is a lot of diarrhea, be sure to give enough of the oral rehydration solution after each stool.
      4) If the infant vomits, keep giving the solution, but give it in sips of 1/2 to 1 teaspoon every few minutes. This will allow time for it to be absorbed. The rate may need to be slower than before the infant vomited.
      5) When people have the correct amount of fluids and salts in their systems, they urinate often and their urine is clear to light yellow in color. If an infant's urine is dark yellow or the infant is not urinating as much as usual, you may wish to give more oral rehydration solution. Call the doctor or clinic if this condition continues.
   c. How to make homemade cereal-based ORS (the sugar is replaced in this solution by the cereal, which is a complex sugar)

Grandma's ORS Recipe

$^1/_2$ to 1 cup of precooked baby rice cereal
2 cups of water
$^1/_4$ teaspoon of table salt

Mix all of the ingredients together until well mixed. Be sure to use a level measuring teaspoon. Make the mixture as thick as is drinkable.

Give it a little at a time, give it often, and give as much as the infant will take. (Give a little every minute if the infant will take it.) You can offer Grandma's ORS with a spoon or a cup. Remember, no gulping. Do not give too much; salt can be dangerous. Remember the idea of replacing fluid: one cup out, one cup in. In other words, the amount of diarrhea that comes out is the amount of fluid that should be put back in.

The ORS solution should be covered and stored in the refrigerator if possible. The solution should be discarded after 6 to 8 hours, or when it is too thick to drink.

Reminder: This is not considered food, and the infant should also be encouraged to eat a normal diet of breast milk, formula, and/or recommended foods.

PARENT EDUCATION PROGRAM: INFANT STIMULATION

Infant stimulation is a program of techniques and tools designed to encourage the growth and development of neonates and infants. Infant stimulation is provided to compensate for the limited opportunities that long-term hospitalized infants have or to augment the activities of an average infant. It is a technique that should be based on the four R's of infant stimulation.

1. Rhythm
   All stimulation techniques should be rhythmical, steady, and unforced.

2. Reciprocity
   All infant stimulation should be reciprocal—should involve interaction, "give and take," between the child and the stimulator. The stimulator must be involved.

3. Repetition
   All infant stimulation activities and techniques should involve repetition to promote better learning, to improve neural pathway development, to provide security, and to maintain goals and skills achieved.

4. Reinforcement
   All infant stimulation activities should provide positive and genuine reinforcement of the worth of the infant as an individual. Reinforcement heightens self-esteem and strengthens the bond and attachment between the infant and the stimulator. The infant and stimulator must approach this as fun time.

Infant stimulation has a profound effect upon the mental, physical, and emotional development of each infant. It enhances the mental development of the infant by stimulating curiosity, cultivating a longer attention span, and promoting more age-appropriate play skills. Infant stimulation affects the physical growth of the infant by promoting better muscle coordination and better muscle control, and infants tend to gain weight faster. Emotionally, infants tend to establish strong attachments, trust that their needs will be met, have a sense of control over their environment, smile sooner and more frequently, are content, and have a secure self-image.

Parents should be encouraged to perform infant stimulation activities. Infant stimulation provided in the home by a consistent caretaker is important to the recently hospitalized infant because these infants receive less individual handling and therefore less stimulation. They are separated from their parents for longer time frames, which interferes with the bonding process and lessens the quality of parent–child interaction. They are often deprived of normal newborn experiences.

The infant stimulation program should be based upon the child's present level of functioning and upon the child's needs along the developmental continuum. Often, a child will be functioning well in the areas of cognition, language, or social/emotional development, yet due to confinement the child's motor skills will be delayed. Therefore, each child's program should be tailored to meet his or her individual needs; it should be based upon the child's developmental age and should provide for activity development in each skill area. Activities selected should encourage age-appropriate play skills while taking into consideration the child's medical situation, developmental age, and capabilities. Infants suspected of delays in any of these areas should be referred to the local early intervention program for evaluation.

Below is a list of suggested play activities and toys for the infant, according to age.

1. 1 month: Provide mobiles, rattles, black-and-white objects, and bright simple pictures lining the crib. The baby enjoys leg/arm cycling and smiles at faces.

2. 2 months: The baby enjoys listening to a variety of sounds, therefore talk and sing to him or her often. Lay the baby on his or her stomach and lay on your stomach with your head facing the baby's. Try to get the baby to hold up his or her head and make eye contact. The baby will also respond to voices.

3. 3 months: Peek-a-boo games encourage discovery. Provide soft, safe, furry cuddle toys. Mount a mirror for the baby.

4. 4 months: Allow some time for the baby to play alone. Encourage movement and rolling. The baby will also react to sounds.

5. 5 months: Provide durable, washable toys with handles. Begin "Pat-a-cake" songs and "So Big" games with gestures. Encourage rocking, wriggling, and rolling by placing objects at arm's length away; this will also encourage the baby to reach out and grab.

6. 6 months: Play "Where's baby?" Play knee games and tummy tickles. The baby will like to laugh and squeal.

7. 7 months: Play hold the baby's hands and encourage standing/walking motion.

8. 8 months: Imitate the baby. Chase the baby. Provide pull toys, stacking blocks, and building blocks.

9. 9 months: The baby will enjoy toys to be picked up with the fingers, push/pull toys, and musical toys.

10. 10 months: Baby books, baby blocks, and children's music are appropriate.

11. 11 months: Riding toys pushed by feet and pop-up toys are suitable.

12. 12 months: Push/pull toys, baby books, children's music, and short videos are appropriate.

PARENT EDUCATION PROGRAM: EMERGENCY CARE GUIDE

Important Numbers

Emergency Medical Services: ______________________________

Poison Control Center: ______________________________

Family Doctor: ______________________________

Bites and Stings

Call 911 (or the local emergency number) immediately if a bite wound is bleeding severely. Proceed as for *Bleeding*, described below. Also do this if the wound is deep or from an unknown animal. If the wound is not bleeding profusely, wash the area with mild soap and running water while you wait for help to arrive, but do not use ointments or creams. If any tissue has been bitten off, wrap it in a clean, wet cloth, place it in a plastic bag, and bring it with you to the hospital. If the child has been stung, call 911 (or the local emergency number) if he or she shows signs of a severe allergic reaction such as shock, wheezing, or spreading rash or welts. This can be life-threatening!!!

Bleeding

Try to control the bleeding by applying direct pressure to the wound or cut with a clean cloth. Elevate the wounded area unless you suspect a broken bone. Call 911 (or the local emergency number) if the bleeding cannot be controlled or if there is a puncture wound caused by a large or embedded object. If the wound seems deep or gaping and you suspect the child needs stitches, go to the hospital emergency room.

Broken Bones and Head/Spine Injuries

In situations such as car accidents, falls greater than the child's height, or significant trauma to the head or spine, assume there is a head or spine injury. Call 911 (or the local emergency number) immediately. Do not move the child; keep him or her still. Control any bleeding (see *Bleeding*, above). For broken bones, immobilize the injured part with a splint—only if you have been properly trained in the technique—and call 911 (or the local emergency number).

Burns

1. If burns are on the child's face, hands, feet, or genitals, or if they are white, blistered, or charred, or larger than the size of the child's hand, call 911 (or the local emergency number). While waiting for paramedics to arrive, cover the burns with a clean, cool, wet towel or sheet, or flush with cool water. For open wounds, use a dry towel.

2. For chemical burns, flush the area with running water until help arrives. Remove any of the child's clothing or jewelry saturated with the chemical as soon as possible.

3. For electrical burns or shock, do not touch the child until you have separated him or her from the power source by turning off the electricity. Check breathing and pulse, then call 911 (or the local emergency number).

4. For minor burns, flush the area with cool water and call the family doctor for follow-up care. Never use ointments, creams, or butter without consulting a physician.

Dental Emergencies

Carefully remove any tooth fragments from the mouth. Do not clean the tooth or remove any tissue attached to it; submerge it in a glass of milk (or water if milk is not available) and take both the child and the tooth to the dentist immediately.

Drowning

Begin cardiopulmonary resuscitation as needed on an unconscious child. If the child's pulse has stopped, have someone call 911 (or the local emergency number) while you begin CPR (see *No Pulse* below).

Poisoning

If the child has any extreme symptoms—such as unconsciousness, breathing difficulties, or seizures—call 911 (or the local emergency number). Otherwise, call the area Poison Control Center, specifying the substance involved, how much was ingested, and the child's age, weight, and condition. Have syrup of ipecac on hand, but do not induce vomiting unless instructed to do so. If you are told to go to a hospital, take the poisonous substance container along.

Any First-Aid Situation (except spine injuries)

After you have given specific care, lay the child on his or her back, elevate the legs slightly, and keep his or her body at a comfortable temperature until help arrives.

Choking

1. Infants up to 12 months
    a. If the baby is coughing forcefully, do not interfere or you may make the situation worse; allow the obstruction to clear itself.
    b. If the infant cannot cough, breathe, or cry:
        1) Stand or sit with him face down along your forearm, resting your arm on your thigh so that the baby's head is lower than his chest; cup his jaw with your hand. With the heel of your other hand, give four quick, firm blows to his back between the shoulder blades.
        2) If this does not dislodge the item, turn the baby onto his back, keeping his head lowered. Give four chest thrusts, with two fingers placed on the breastbone one finger's-width below the imaginary line connecting the nipples. Compress the breastbone 1/2 to 1 inch with each thrust.
        3) Repeat the combination of back blows and chest thrusts until the object comes out or until the infant becomes unconscious In either case, have the baby checked later for internal injuries.

   c. If the infant loses consciousness, roll the infant onto his or her back; avoid twisting the body and neck. Open the airway by tilting the head back gently. Push down on the forehead until the chin points up and the mouth drops open.

2. Children 12 months and older

   a. If the child is coughing forcefully, talking, or breathing, don't do anything; allow the obstruction to clear itself.

   b. For a conscious child who cannot breathe at all, perform the Heimlich maneuver. Bring your arms around the child from behind. Make a fist, and place the thumb side against the middle of the abdomen just above the navel. Grab your fist with your other hand and press in with quick, upward thrusts. Repeat until the object comes out or the child becomes unconscious.

   c. If the child loses consciousness:

      1) Roll the child onto his or her back; avoid twisting the neck and back. Open the airway by tilting the head back gently. Push down on the forehead while lifting the chin. Look, listen, and feel breathing for 3 to 5 seconds. If the child shows no sign of breathing, pinch the nose shut and cover the mouth with yours. Blow in two puffs of air, taking a breath in between. Watch the chest as you do this; if it does not rise, re-tilt the head and do it again.

      2) If the chest still does not rise, administer blows and thrusts as for *Choking*, above. Then do a foreign-object check. Open the mouth, holding the tongue down with your thumb. If you can see an object (and only if you can see one), remove it by sweeping your little finger with a hook action along the base of the tongue. Repeat the cycle of head-tilt/chin-lift, two breaths, blows and thrusts, and object check until breaths go in.

      3) If breaths do go in, check for a pulse for 5 to 10 seconds with two fingers placed on the inside of the child's upper arm midway between the elbow and the armpit. If there is a pulse, but still no breathing, continue breathing into the mouth and nose once every 3 seconds. If you cannot detect a pulse within 10 seconds, start CPR (see *No Pulse*, below).

No Pulse

1. If the infant is not breathing and has no pulse, give CPR. Place two fingers on the breastbone, one finger's-width below the nipple line. Push the chest downward 1/2 to 1 inch and release, five times in quick succession (within 3 seconds). Then give one breath (as in *Choking*, item 2.c.1, above). Continue CPR for 1 minute, then recheck the pulse. If there is no pulse, give one rescue breath and continue CPR until the pulse resumes or help arrives.

2. When breaths do go in, check for a pulse on the side of the neck. If there is a pulse but still no breathing, continue breathing into the mouth once every 4 seconds. If you cannot detect a pulse within 10 seconds, start CPR.

Unconsciousness and Choking

Give 6 to 10 quick upward thrusts with the heel of your hand placed just above the navel. Then open the mouth, holding the tongue down with your thumb; if you can see a foreign object, remove it by sweeping your little finger with a hook action along the base of the tongue. Repeat the cycle of head-tilt/chin-lift, two breaths, blows and thrusts, and object check until breaths go in (as in *Choking*, item 2.c.1, above).

PARENT EDUCATION PROGRAM: BASIC HOME SAFETY

Fire Safety (to eliminate fire hazards)

1. The furnace and water heater should be checked at least once a year to ensure safety.
2. Wood stoves or portable heaters should be installed properly, and chimneys should be cleaned and inspected once a year.
3. Flammable liquids should be stored outside, away from any heat source, and disposed of properly.
4. Electrical appliances should be used safely and checked periodically.
5. Matches, cigarettes, and smoking materials should be disposed of safely in an ashtray or fire-resistant container.
6. The kitchen stove should be kept free of grease. No loose-fitting clothes should be worn when cooking. Pot handles should be turned away from the front of the stove and potholders always should be used.
7. Oxygen should be used away from open flames and heat. Do not place concentrator near a heat source. Tubing should not come in contact with stoves, space heaters, or baseboard heating coils. Do not use electrical devices, such as electric razors, while using oxygen. Post "NO SMOKING" signs. Clean up any oil or grease before using oxygen (as it may combine with oxygen and spontaneously ignite).
8. Develop a fire safety plan.
   a. Standard fire regulations recommend one smoke detector on every level of the home.
   b. Develop an evacuation plan for use in case of fire. Note which family members will require assistance because of age, illness, or disability.
   c. Establish clear pathways to all exits. Do not block exits with furniture or boxes.
   d. Have keys stored near doors locked with deadbolts.
   e. Do not leave cooking unattended for long periods of time.
   f. Chimneys should be inspected annually to avoid dangerous buildup of creosote.
   g. Kerosene heaters, wood stoves, and fireplaces should not be left unattended while in use. Never use a gas stove for space heating.
   h. Have a fire extinguisher in an easily accessible place (e.g., kitchen).

Electrical Safety

1. Cords must not be placed beneath furniture or rugs.
2. Replace frayed cords.
3. Do not overload extension cords. Check rating labels on cords and appliances.
4. Multiple outlet adapters should not be used on electrical outlets.

5. Cover unused outlets, and teach young children not to touch plugs, cords, or outlets.
6. Never replace a fuse with a penny or a higher amp fuse. Use correctly sized fuses at all times.
7. Never turn on an appliance or plug one in while standing in water or if your hands are wet.
8. Call a professional electrician if you suspect an electrical problem. Blown fuses or dimmed lights may indicate a wiring problem.
9. Make sure the electrical system is sufficient when using medical equipment such as ventilators and oxygen concentrators. Check with the medical supplier or an electrician.
10. Use three-pronged adapters when required.
11. When ambulating with a pump, IV pole, electrical cord, or IV tubing, carefully position the equipment between you and the outlet, to avoid falls or electrical accidents.

Environmental Safety

1. Loose rugs, runners, and mats should be secured to the floor with double-sided tape or rubber matting.
2. Carpet edges should be tacked down.
3. Torn, worn, frayed carpeting should be repaired, replaced, or removed.
4. Cupboards should be organized so that frequently used items are on lower shelves.
5. A sturdy stepstool should be used to reach items on high shelves.
6. Heavy items should be stored flat on lower levels of the closet to avoid falls and injury.
7. Stairs, hallways, and passageways between rooms should be well lit and free of clutter.
8. Stairs should have sturdy, well-secured handrails on both sides. Install gates, if needed, to protect children from falls.
9. Avoid using stairs while wearing only socks or smooth-soled shoes.
10. Furniture should be arranged to allow free movement in heavy traffic areas.
11. Hazardous tools and firearms should be kept locked up. Unplug appliances and tools when not in use.
12. Cleaning fluids, polishes, bleaches, detergents, and all poisons should be stored separately and clearly marked. Proper ventilation should be available when cleaning fluids are being used.
13. Spills should be cleaned up promptly.
14. Old newspapers and cleaning cloths should not be stockpiled.
15. Insects, rodents, and bad odors should be controlled.

16. Place at least one phone in a position that is accessible in the event that an accident renders a person unable to stand. Emergency numbers should be posted near the phone, including ambulance, doctor, fire, police, and poison control.

17. Entrance ways should be clear of leaves, snow, and ice.

Bathroom Safety

1. Tubs and showers should have a textured surface or nonskid mats or strips to prevent falls.

2. Grab-bars to assist transfers should be installed in tub, showers, and toilet areas when applicable.

3. Check the water temperature with your hand before entering the tub or shower. The water temperature setting may need to be lowered.

4. A night light should be used in the bathroom if possible.

5. A bell, buzzer, or appropriate noisemaker should be placed in the bathroom for emergency use.

6. Ground fault outlets should be installed.

7. Electrical appliances should be used away from water.

8. The door lock should be a type that can be opened from the outside in an emergency.

9. Never leave a child alone in the bathtub. ***A child can drown in a few inches of water!!!***

10. If possible, locate a bathroom on the first floor.

Bibliography

Alaska Department of Health and Social Services: *Alaska Maternal and Child Health Manual for Public Health Nursing.* Alaska Department of Health and Social Services, Division of Public Health, Section of Nursing, Anchorage, Alaska; June 1994.

American Diabetes Association: *Medical Management of Pregnancy Complicated by Diabetes.* American Diabetes Association, Alexandria, Virginia; 1993.

Arkin, Elaine Bratic, and Judith E. Funkhouser: *Communicating About Alcohol and Other Drugs: Strategies for Reaching Populations at Risk.* U.S. Department of Public Health and Human Services, Rockville, Maryland; 1990.

Association of Maternal and Child Health Programs: *Caring for Mothers and Children. A Report of a Survey of FY 1987 State MCH Program Activities.* Association of Maternal and Child Health Programs, Washington, D.C.; March 1989.

Association of Maternal and Child Health Programs: *Toward the Future of Title V! A Report on Site Visits to Ten State Programs.* Association of Maternal and Child Health Programs, Washington, D.C.; November 1991.

Association of Maternal and Child Health Programs: *Meeting Needs, Building Capacities. State Perspectives on Graduate Training and Continuing Education Needs of Title V Programs.* Association of Maternal and Child Health Programs, Washington, D.C.; October 1992.

Association of Women's Health, Obstetric, and Neonatal Nurses: *Practice Resource: Preparation for Technology-Dependent Infants.* Association of Women's Health, Obstetric, and Neonatal Nurses, McLean VA; January 1993.

Bass, Alison: Few support services are available once ill children go home. *Boston Sunday Globe,* November 27, 1988.

Betz, Cecily Lynn, et al.: Altered digestive function. *Family Centered Nursing Care of Infants,* 35:1478–1480; 1994.

Block, Carol, et al.: *Home Care for High-Risk Infants, The First Year. Caring,* pp. 11–17. National Association for Home Care, Washington, D.C.; May 1989.

Boland, Mary G., and Lynn Czarniecki: Starting life with HIV, *RN,* pp. 54–58; January 1991.

Bradley, Robert, and Bettye Caldwell: Using the HOME inventory to assess the family environment. *Pediatric Nursing,* 14(2):97–102; March–April 1988.

Briggs, Nancy: Hospitals & home care: Inseparable in the '80's. *Pediatric Nursing,* 12(5):384–385; September–October 1986.

Briggs, Nancy, Connie Lierman, Julie Hazelton, Richard Wolff, Kinny Pasquera, and Elizabeth Wilson: Multidisciplinary treatment of feeding disorders in the home. *Pediatric Nursing,* 13(4):266–271; July–August 1987.

Britton, John R., and Helen Britton: Efficacy of early newborn discharge in a middle-class population. *MDC,* 138:1041–1045; November 1984.

Britton, John R., Helen Britton, and Susan Beebe: Early discharge of the term newborn: A continued dilemma. *Pediatrics,* 94(3):291–295; September 1994.

Brown, Sarah S., ed.: *Prenatal Care. Reaching Mothers. Reaching Infants.* National Academy Press, Washington, D.C.; 1988.

Boyer, D.: Prediction of postpartum depression. *NAACOG Clinical Issues in Perinatal and Women's Health Nursing,* 1(3):267–278; 1990.

Casey, Robert P.: *Investing in Our Children and Families, 1993–94 Budget Initiatives*. Executive Office, Harrisburg, Pennsylvania; 1993.

Casey, Robert P.: *Managed Competition: A Health Care System for Pennsylvania*. Report of the Pennsylvania Economic Development Partnership Health Care Committee to The Pennsylvania Economic Development Partnership. Executive Office, Harrisburg, Pennsylvania; November 1992.

Child Health Foundation: Diarrhea kills over 300 U.S. children annually. *NEWS, Child Health Foundation Newsletter*, Columbia, Maryland; June 2, 1996.

Children's Hospital of Los Angeles: *Informational Guidelines for Parents*. Children's Hospital of Los Angeles, Nutrition Support Program, Los Angeles; 1990.

Children's Hospital of Philadelphia: *Informational Guidelines for Parents*. Children's Hospital of Philadelphia, Nutrition Support Program, Philadelphia; 1991.

Commonwealth of Pennsylvania, Department of Health: *Maternal and Child Health Services*. Draft Block Grant Application, Federal Fiscal Year 1993. Pennsylvania Department of Health, Harrisburg, Pennsylvania; 1993.

Commonwealth of Pennsylvania, Department of Health: *Guide to Health Data for Pennsylvania*. State Health Data Center, Harrisburg, Pennsylvania; June 1996.

Commonwealth of Pennsylvania, Department of Public Welfare: *Pennsylvania Medical Assistance Program Eligibility Verification System Manual*. Publication 261. Pennsylvania Department of Public Welfare, Harrisburg, Pennsylvania; April 1993.

Commonwealth of Pennsylvania, Department of Public Welfare: Statistics provided by outpatient staff. Pennsylvania Department of Public Welfare, Harrisburg, Pennsylvania; May 13, 1993.

Commonwealth of Pennsylvania, Department of Public Welfare: *Overview, The Family Care Network*. Pennsylvania Department of Public Welfare, Harrisburg, Pennsylvania; 1994.

Cook, Paddy, Robert Petersen, and Dorothy Moore: *Alcohol, Tobacco, and Other Drugs May Harm the Newborn*. United States Department of Health and Human Services, Rockville, Maryland; 1990.

Cornelius, Llewellyn B.: Barriers to medical care for white, black, and Hispanic American children. *Journal of the National Medical Association*, 85(4):281–288; 1993.

Corporation for Public Broadcasting: *Miracle of Life*. Video production airing on public broadcasting series NOVA. Corporation for Public Broadcasting, Films for Humanities and Sciences, Monmouth Junction, New Jersey; 1983.

Craven, Ruth F.: *Fundamentals of Nursing*, 2nd edition. Lippincott–Raven Publishers, Philadelphia; 1996.

Cunningham, Gary, and Marshall Lindheimer: Hypertension in pregnancy. *New England Journal of Medicine*, 326(14):927–931; 1992.

Davis, Matthew, ed.: *Health Care Reform Update*, 1(8). National Association for Home Care; Washington, D.C.; May 12, 1993.

Dingell, John D., and Committee of Conference: *Conference Report, ADAMNA Reorganization Act. Title V. Home Visiting Services for At-Risk Families*. 102nd Congress, 2nd Session, House of Representatives, Report 102-546. U.S. House of Representatives, Washington, D.C.; 1994.

Donar, Mary: Community care: Pediatric home mechanical ventilation. *Holistic Nursing Practice*, 2(2):68–80; 1988.

Falkner, F., ed.: *Prevention of Infant Mortality and Morbidity. Child Health and Development*, Volume 4. Karger, Basel, Switzerland; 1985.

Farber, Anne E.: *Survey of Home Visiting Programs for Children and Families in Pennsylvania, Executive Summary*. University of Pittsburgh, University Center for Social and Urban Reseach, Office of Child Development, Pittsburgh, Pennsylvania; 1996.

Fitzgerald, Susan: 1 in 6 New mothers used cocaine, study finds. *Philadelphia Inquirer*; April 8, 1989.

Fitzgerald, Susan: How three nations shape birth. *Philadelphia Inquirer, Suburban Edition*; April 27, 1993.

Friesen, Barbara J., Joanne Griesbach, Judith Jacobs, Judith Katz-Leavy, and Dennis Olson: Improving services for families. *Children Today*, pp. 18–22; July–August 1988.

Federal Register: Medicare regulations. *Federal Register: Rules and Regulations*, 54(153); August 14, 1989.

Fleming, Barbara W.: Assessing and promoting positive parenting in adolescent mothers. *MCN*, 18:32–37; January–February 1993.

Grabert, B., C. Wardell, and S. Harburg: Home phototherapy. *Clinical Pediatrics*, 25:291–294; 1986.

Harrison, H., and A. Kositsky: *The Premature Baby Book*. St. Martin's Press, New York; 1983.

Henrikson, Mary, Ginna Wall, Dona Lethbridge, and Vicki McClurg: Nursing diagnosis and obstetric, gynecologic, and neonatal nursing: Breastfeeding as an example. *JOGN Thoughts and Opinions*, 21(6); November–December 1992.

Herman, Robin: France wants me to have this baby. *Washington Post*; May 1, 1990.

Hoerlin, Bettina Yaffe: *Targeting for the Future: Health Care in the Philadelphia Region*. Report to The Pew Charitable Trusts, Philadelphia, Pennsylvania; January 1989.

Howard, Tracy: *Kids Ending Hunger. What Can We Do?* Andrews and McMeel, A Universal Press Syndicate Co., Kansas City, Missouri; 1992.

Hyde-Robertson, Barbara L.: The necessity for maternal–infant perinatal home care. *Caring*, pp. 26–31. National Association for Home Care, Washington, D.C.; December 1992.

Infante-Rivard, Claire, Gisele Filion, Mona Baumgarten, Madeleine Bourassa, Johanne Labelle, and Monique Messier: A public health home intervention among families of low socioeconomic status. *CHC*, 18(2):102; Spring 1989.

Institute of Medicine: *Nutrition During Pregnancy and Lactation*. National Academy Press, Washington, D.C.; 1990.

Johns Hopkins Oral Rehydration Project: *Outpatient Oral Rehydration Therapy Protocol*. Johns Hopkins Oral Rehydration Project, Baltimore, Maryland; 1991.

Johnson, S., and D. Kraut: *Pregnancy and Bedrest: A Guide for the Pregnant Woman and Her Family*. St. Martin's Press, New York; 1990.

Langevin, Jeanne: Using home health aids in a high-risk infant program. *Caring*, pp. 40–43. National Association for Home Care, Washington, D.C.; June 1988.

Marecki, Marsha: Postpartum followup goals and assessment. *JOGN*, pp. 214–218; August 1979.

Marks, Margaret G.: *Introductory Pediatric Nursing*, 4th edition. Lippincott–Raven Publishers, Philadelphia; 1994.

McAnarney, Elizabeth R.: Experience with an adolescent health care program. *Public Health Reports*, 90(5):412–416; September–October 1975.

McAnarney, Elizabeth R.: Development of an adolescent maternity project in Rochester, New York. *Public Health Reports*, 92(2):154–159; March–April 1977.

NAACOG: *Criteria Established for Identifying At-Risk Infants*, 14(10). NAACOG, Washington, D.C.; October 1987.

NAACOG: *OGN Nursing Practice Resource: Neonatal Skin Care*. NAACOG, Washington, D.C.; 1992.

National Center for Education in Maternal and Child Health: *Reaching Out: A Directory of National Organizations Related to Maternal and Child Health*. National Center for Education in Maternal and Child Health, Washington, D.C.; March 1989.

Nettina, Sandra M.: *Lippincott Manual of Nursing Practice*, 6th edition. Lippincott–Raven Publishers, Philadelphia; 1996.

North Carolina Department of Health: *MCH Manual*. Department of Public Health, Durham, North Carolina; 1992.

Nuttal, P.: Maternal responses to home apnea monitoring of infants. *Nursing Research*, 37:354–357; 1988.

Oehler, Jerri N., et al.: How to target infants at highest risk for developmental delay. *Maternal–Child Nursing*, 18:20–23; January–February 1993.

Olds, D.: The prenatal/infancy project: A strategy for responding to the needs of high risk mothers and their children. *Prevention in Human Services*, 7(1):59–87; 1989.

Olds, D., C. Henderson, R. Tatlebaum, and R. Chamberlin: Improving the delivery of prenatal care and outcomes of pregnancy: A randomized trial of nurse home visitation. *Pediatrics*, 77(1):16–28; January 1986.

Olds, D., and H. Kitzman: Can home visitation improve the health of women and children at environmental risk? *Pediatrics*, 1(1):108–116; July 1990.

Pennsylvania Department of Health: *Block Grant, Commonwealth of Pennsylvania Preventive and Primary Care Services for Pregnant Women, Mothers, and Infants up to Age 1, Component A*, p. 64. Pennsylvania Department of Health, Division of Maternal Child Health, Harrisburg, Pennsylvania.

Pennsylvania Department of Health: *Vital Statistics 1990*. Pennsylvania Department of Health, State Health Data Center, Harrisburg, Pennsylvania; 1992.

Pennsylvania Healthy Mothers, Healthy Babies Coalition: *Pennsylvania Healthy Mothers, Healthy Babies Coalition* Pennsylvania Healthy Mothers, Healthy Babies Coalition, Bryn Mawr, Pennsylvania; 1992.

Pennsylvania Partnerships for Children: *Our Children, Our Future.* Breakfast on Children's Health Issues. Pennsylvania Partnerships for Children, Harrisburg, Pennsylvania; October 9, 1991.

Pennsylvania Partnerships for Children: *Kids Count.* State Grant Proposal for Pennsylvania. Pennsylvania Partnerships for Children, Harrisburg, Pennsylvania; August 13, 1992.

Perrin, James M.: Chronically ill children, in America, the case for home care. *Journal for Physicians in Home Care;* Spring 1987.

Philadelphia Department of Public Health: *Selected Resident Birth and Death Data by Health District, by Census Tract and by Neighborhood, 1983–1993.* Department of Public Health, Philadelphia, 1994.

Reece, S.: Social support and the early maternal experience for primiparas over 35. *Maternal–Child Nursing Journal,* 3:91–98; July–September 1993.

Reeder, S., L. Martin, and D. Koniak-Griffin: *Maternity Nursing, Family Newborn and Women's Health Care,* 18th edition. Lippincott–Raven Publishers, Philadelphia; 1997.

Richmond, Frederick, Martha Wade Steketee, et al.: *The State of the Child: A Profile of Pennsylvania's Children.* Waldman Graphics, Philadelphia; 1993.

Roberts, Joyce: Current perspectives in preeclampsia. *Journal of Nurse Midwifery,* 39(2):70–90; 1994.

Rogatz, Peter: Perspective on home care. *Public Health Nursing,* 4(1):7–8; March 1987.

Rosen, C., D. Glaze, and J. Frost: Home monitor followup of persistent apnea and bradycardia in preterm infants. *American Journal of Diseases in Children,* 140:547–550; 1986.

Shelton, Terri I., Elizabeth Jeppson, and Beverly Johnson: *Family Centered Care for Children with Special Health Care Needs,* 2nd edition. Association for the Care of Children's Health, U.S. Public Health Service, Division of Maternal Child Health, Rockville, Maryland; 1987.

Sills, Joanne: Infant deaths soar in areas. *Philadelphia Daily News;* July 8, 1992.

Sirkka, L.: Health promotion in child and family health care: The role of the Finnish public health nurses. *Public Health Nursing,* 11(1):32–37; February 1994.

Smith, Judy: The dangers of prenatal cocaine use. *Maternal–Child Nursing,* 13:174–179; May–June 1992.

South Carolina Department of Health and Environmental Control: *Comprehensive Risk Screening for Patient Referrals.* South Carolina Department of Health and Environmental Control, Maternal Health, Columbia, South Carolina; October 1992.

Stanwick, Richard S., Michael E. K. Moffat, Yvonne Robitaille, Aline Edmond, and Caroline Dok: An evaluation of the routine postnatal public health nurse home visit. *Canadian Journal of Public Health,* 73:200–205; May–June 1982.

Starn, J.: Community health nursing visits for at risk women and infants. *Journal of Community Health Nursing,* 9(2):103–110; 1992.

Streeter, N. S.: Discharge planning home care. *Journal of Perinatal and Neonatal Nursing* 5(1); 1991.

Sullivan, Joan, et al.: Can we help the substance abusing mother and infant? *Maternal–Child Nursing,* 18:153–157; May–June 1993.

United Way of Pennsylvania: *Report of the Success-By-Six Coalition: Helping All Children Succeed for Life.* United Way of Pennsylvania, Harrisburg, Pennsylvania; June 1992.

U.S.D.L., Occupational Safety and Health, Office of Health Compliance Assistance: *OSHA Instruction CPL 2-2, 44A,* p. 4. U.S. Department of Labor Occupational Safety and Health, Office of Health Compliance Assistance, Washington, D.C.; August 15, 1988.

U.S.D.P.H., Agency for Health Care Policy and Research: *The 50 Most Frequent Diagnosis-Related Groups (DRO's), Diagnoses, and Procedures: Statistics by Hospital Size and Location.* Hospital Studies Program Research Note 13. U.S. Department of Public Health, Agency for Health Care Policy and Research, Rockville, Maryland; September 1990.

U.S.D.P.H., Agency for Health Care Policy and Research: *Research Activities: Contracts Awarded for Low Birthweight, Health Care for Women, Barriers to Quality Care Persist.* Publication No. 158. U.S. Department of Public Health, Agency for Health Care Policy and Research, Rockville, Maryland; November 1992.

U.S.D.P.H., Agency for Health Care Policy and Research: *Research Activities: Number of Uninsured Children on the Rise, Less than 15 Percent of America's Health Care Dollar Spent on Children.* Publication No. 162. U.S. Department of Public Health, Agency for Health Care Policy and Research, Rockville, Maryland; March 1993.

U.S.D.P.H., Agency for Health Care Policy and Research: *Research Activities: Women Planning Pregnancy*

Often Switch to HMO's. Publication No. 163. U.S. Department of Public Health, Agency for Health Care Policy and Research, Rockville, Maryland; April 1993.

U.S.D.P.H., Agency for Health Care Policy and Research: *Research Activities: Uninsured Patients More Likely to Die Prematurely*. Publication No. 169. U.S. Department of Public Health, Agency for Health Care Policy and Research, Rockville, Maryland; October 1993.

U.S.D.P.H., Agency for Health Care Policy and Research: *Research Activities: Financially Troubled Hospitals Face Difficult Choices, Outlook Poor for Very Young Babies with AIDS, Teen Health Programs Often Deficient in On Site Services*. Publication No. 170. U.S. Department of Public Health, Agency for Health Care Policy and Research, Rockville, Maryland; November 1993.

U.S.D.P.H.H.S.: *Caring for Our Future: The Content of Prenatal Care*. U.S. Department of Public Health and Human Services, Washington, D.C.; 1989.

Vrazo, Fawn: Pregnant doctors in distress. *Philadelphia Inquirer*; February 17, 1990.

Vrazo, Fawn: Lying in is now out for many new mothers. *Philadelphia Inquirer*; August 17, 1990.

Vrazo, Fawn: Lying in is out as insurers cut post-childbirth coverage. *Philadelphia Inquirer*; August 7, 1993.

Wasik, B., D. Bryant, and C. Lyons: *Home Visiting: Procedures for Helping Families*. Sage Publications, Newbury Park, California; 1990.

Weston, Donna R., Barbara Ivins, Barry Zuckerman, Coryl Jones, and Richard Lopez: *Drug Exposed Babies: Research and Clinical Issues*. National Center for Clinical Infant Programs, Washington, D.C.; June 1989.

Williams, Lenore, and Mary Cooper: Nurse managed postpartum home care. *JOGN Principles and Practice*, pp. 25–31; January–February 1993.

Wisconsin Association for Perinatal Care: *Early Discharge—Short Term Length of Stay*. Wisconsin Association for Perinatal Care; June 1993.

Yariover, Mark J., Deloras Jones, and Michael D. Miller: Perinatal care of low risk mothers and infants. *New England Journal of Medicine*, 294(13):702–705; March 25, 1976.

Young, L., D. Creighton, and R. Sauve: The needs of families of infants discharged home with continous oxygen therapy. *Journal of Obstetric, Gynecolgic, and Neonatal Nursing*, 17:187–193; 1987.

Zuravin, Susan J.: *Child Maltreatment and Teenage First Births: A Relationship Mediated by Chronic Sociodemographic Stress?* American Orthopsychiatric Association, Washington, D.C.; January 1988.

Additional Resources

Free or low-cost educational material can be obtained from the following additional health information resources.

U.S. Department of Health and Human Services
Public Health Service Office of Disease Prevention and Health Promotion
ONHIC, P.O. Box 1133
Washington, DC 20013-1133
(800) 336-4797
Request the *Health Information Resources Catalogue*

Maternal Child Health Bureau
March of Dimes Birth Defects Foundation
National Center for Education in Maternal Child Health
Write to: National Maternal Child Health Clearing House
8201 Greensboro Drive, Suite 600
McLean, VA 22102
(703) 821-8955, ext. 254 or 265
Request *Prenatal Care, A Resource Guide*

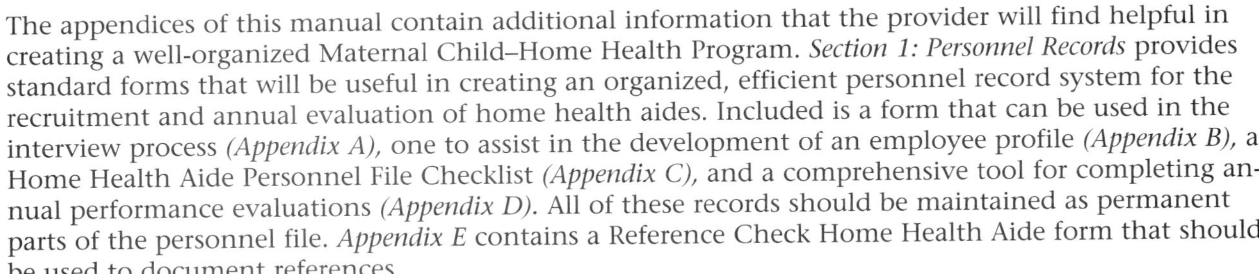

Appendices

The appendices of this manual contain additional information that the provider will find helpful in creating a well-organized Maternal Child–Home Health Program. *Section 1: Personnel Records* provides standard forms that will be useful in creating an organized, efficient personnel record system for the recruitment and annual evaluation of home health aides. Included is a form that can be used in the interview process *(Appendix A),* one to assist in the development of an employee profile *(Appendix B),* a Home Health Aide Personnel File Checklist *(Appendix C),* and a comprehensive tool for completing annual performance evaluations *(Appendix D).* All of these records should be maintained as permanent parts of the personnel file. *Appendix E* contains a Reference Check Home Health Aide form that should be used to document references.

The objective of any training program is to assure that persons providing care are competent. Therefore, an integral component in training must include a means of measuring competency. Persons working in home care must be able to function much more independently than those working within an institution where supervisory help is always on site. *Section 2: Competency Tests* provides tests that should be given as part of the training program *(Appendix F).* It is crucial that all persons be tested by both oral and written means, as well as through direct supervision of actual client care, to determine their competency prior to working independently. Competency testing is a requirement of the federal Medicare program for Home Health Aides and the Joint Commission on the Accreditation of Healthcare Organizations (JCAHO) and the National League of Nursing (NLN). Copies of all competency evaluations and tests should be maintained as a permanent part of the personnel file.

Section 3: Clinical Records provides the required clinical records for a Home Health Aide program seeking Medicare certification, or accreditation through JCAHO or NLN. Organizations other than home care agencies offering paraprofessional services will also find these helpful in creating a program that offers a means of monitoring and documenting quality of care. Included is a copy of the standard Plan of Care developed for use by the Health Care Financing Administration (HCFA; *Appendix G).* This document records the physician orders for home care services and should be completed by the supervising nurse and shared with the home health aide. Also included are clinical records to be used by the nurse in developing a comprehensive plan for Home Health Aide services as well as by professionals in other disciplines such as physical therapy and social work. Included in addition to the HCFA form are the following.

1. **Home Health Client Rights and Consent Forms:** Organizations will want to modify this form to assure that clients have the hotline phone number to their individual state surveyor office. For Medicare certified agencies, allowing clients access to this number is a federal requirement. *(See Appendices H–J.)*
2. **Initial Evaluation Form:** This is to be completed by the nurse as part of the medical assessment on the first visit. This includes the Current Medication Profile, to be completed by the nurse at the first visit and updated at each subsequent visit. Although aides do not administer medications, they should be familiar with them in order to have a fuller understanding of the the client's needs. *(See Appendix K.)*
3. **Pediatric Assessment and Care Screening Tool:** This determines functional limitations. This form was designed to measure functional ability in the infant/child. It should be completed by the nurse at the first visit and will be used to assist in determining developmental delays that interfere with the infant/child's performance of age-appropriate activities of daily living. *(See Appendix L.)*

The concept for this assessment was derived as a result of the author's involvement with the Federal Uniform Needs Assessment Task Force during the development of the Uniform Needs Assessment Tool currently used in the Medicare program to assess adult functional ability in the performance of activities of daily living. A 65-year-old previously healthy adult now unable to walk due to a stroke is considered functionally impaired and in need of rehabilitation. Home Health Aide support is accessible through Medicare to assist with the performance of activities of daily living such as ambulating, bathing, and feeding, which the client would be able to do independently without the functional impairment.

Children, though, cannot be measured with this Uniform Needs Assessment Tool because functional appropriateness for a child has to be measured against expectations for the age. It is functionally normal for a 9-month-old not to walk, but it is not normal for a 9-month-old to have inadequate muscle development and strength to sit independently. This child requires assistance to perform a functional activity that by 9 months should be done independently. Functional Assessments for a child must assess age-appropriate development. Pediatric researchers Stein and Jessop recognized the deficits in measuring the functional ability of children and developed their own tool that was studied intensely.

The tool in this manual provides an objective means of assessing age-appropriate functional ability in infants and children. Based upon deficits found or areas of concern, the nurse should develop a comprehensive plan to be shared with all care providers and to assist in the development of a Home Health Aide Care Plan that will focus on working with and improving functional deficits, if possible.*

4. **Nursing Plan of Care and Progress Record:** This is to be used by the nurse for subsequent home visits. *(See Appendix M.)*
5. **Supervisory Note:** This should be completed by the nurse at each visit to provide home health aide supervision. *(See Appendix N.)*
6. **Home Health Aide Care Plan:** Developed by the nurse for the home health aide to follow in the provision of care. Developed based on the needs found in the initial evaluation which includes a medical and functional assessment. *(See Appendix O.)*
7. **Home Health Aide Clinical Record:** This is to be completed by the aide. Performance should parallel the direction given in the Home Health Aide Care Plan. *(See Appendix P.)*
8. **Nursing Progress Notes:** This is for use by nurses and aides. Home health aides should summarize care for each visit or shift. *(See Appendix Q.)*
9. **Pediatric Intake and Output:** A clinical record tool the nurse may find helpful to have the client's family and the aide maintain. It should be reviewed by the nurse on each visit. *(See Appendix R.)*
10. **Discharge Summary:** This is to be completed by the nurse at the end of care. *(See Appendix S.)*

Section 4: Basic Policies and Procedures, deals with vital signs and contains outlines of procedures that can distributed to the home health aides. *(See Appendix T.)*

The Bibiliography preceding the Appendices will be useful in developing a resource library. The manual concludes with a list of Abbreviations, a helpful Glossary, and a detailed Index.

*The author wishes to acknowledge the work of the Federal Task Force responsible for developing the Uniform Needs Assessment Tool and Doctors Ruth Stein and Dorothy Jessop for their recognition of the need to apply uniform needs assessment to infants and children.

Appendix **A**

Home Health Aide Interview Form

Name: ______________________ Date of interview: ______________________

Interviewer: ______________________

Title: ______________________

Personal appearance: ______________________

Communication skills: ______________________

Interests:

Experience related to agency needs: ______________________

Strengths:

Areas of concern to applicant: ______________________

Summary:

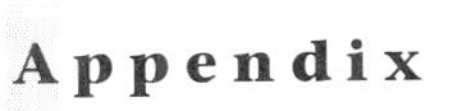
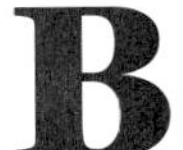

Appendix B

Home Health Aide Profile

Name: ______________________ Starting date: ______________________

Address: ____

Phone: ______________________ Other phone: ______________________

In case of emergency, please notify: ______________________ phone: ______________

Certificate: ____

No. of hours: ____________ Ped/OB hours: ____________

Training needed: HHA complete ______ HHA—OB/Ped ______

Probation period: from ______________ to ______________

Probation review completed by: ______________________ date: ______________

First 1000 hours performance review

Due: ______________________

Completed: ______________ by: ______________________

Work preference profile

Case type: ____ Peds ____ Neo ____ OB ____ Other

Shift: ____ 7–3 ____ 3–11 ____ 11–7

Part time: ____ < 20 hours ____ > 20 hours

Full time: ____ Mon–Fri only ____ Sun/Sat inclusive ____ Holidays ____ Weekends

Special schedule (detail): ______________________

Geographic preference: ______________________

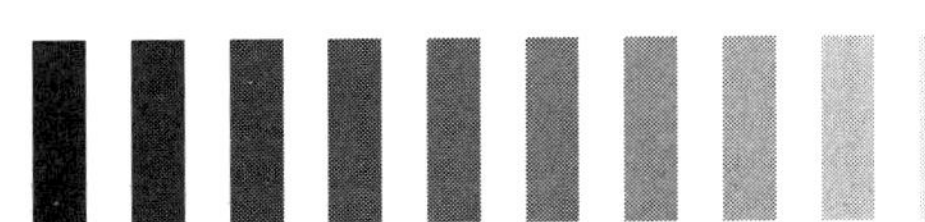

Appendix **C**

Home Health Aide Personnel File Checklist

All Home Health Aides must have the following in their personnel file and keep the dated information current. (Dated items are marked with ***.)

To be completed and maintained in personnel file.

Interview Form _______

Completed Application _______

Employment Aggreement _______

Employment Status Form _______

Completed Profile _______

W-4 IRS Form*** _______

Physical Examination*** _______

Criminal Record Form _______

Two References _______

CPR Certification*** _______

HHA Certification _______

Auto Insurance _______ Optional

Performance Review*** _______ Annual

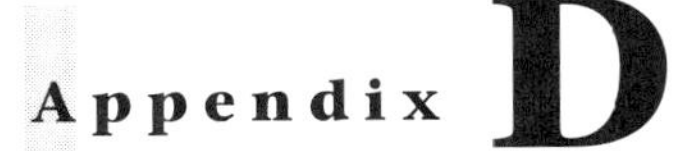

Appendix D

Home Health Aide Performance Review

Name: ______________________________

Employment start date: _______________

Review date: _______________

Reviewer: ______________________________

Supervisor: ______________________________

Indicate to what extent Home Health Aide fulfills principal function: least = 1, most = 5.

Provides assistance to clients to achieve maximum self-reliance	1	2	3	4	5
Preparation of nutritious meals	1	2	3	4	5
Supports client through difficult events	1	2	3	4	5
Maintains clean, healthful environment	1	2	3	4	5
Reports changes in client condition	1	2	3	4	5

Home Health Aide: ______________________ Date: ____________

Indicate level of performance of responsibility

Accepts case	Poor	Fair	Good	Very Good	Excellent
Takes supervision	Poor	Fair	Good	Very Good	Excellent
Participates in developing care plan	Poor	Fair	Good	Very Good	Excellent
Implements care plan	Poor	Fair	Good	Very Good	Excellent
Relates to client/family	Poor	Fair	Good	Very Good	Excellent
Teaches client/family	Poor	Fair	Good	Very Good	Excellent
Performs procedures	Poor	Fair	Good	Very Good	Excellent
Assists client in transition	Poor	Fair	Good	Very Good	Excellent
Client care and management	Poor	Fair	Good	Very Good	Excellent
Prepares meals	Poor	Fair	Good	Very Good	Excellent
Performs household tasks	Poor	Fair	Good	Very Good	Excellent
Observes/reports safety hazards	Poor	Fair	Good	Very Good	Excellent
Maintains communication with supervisor	Poor	Fair	Good	Very Good	Excellent
Documents appropriately and accurately	Poor	Fair	Good	Very Good	Excellent
Maintains confidentiality	Poor	Fair	Good	Very Good	Excellent
Follows through correctly on agency policies	Poor	Fair	Good	Very Good	Excellent

Indicate compliance level

Home Health Aide is prompt	Seldom	Sometimes	Usually	Always
Home Health Aide is neat and professional	Seldom	Sometimes	Usually	Always
Home Health Aide continues learning	Seldom	Sometimes	Usually	Always
Home Health Aide is conscientious	Seldom	Sometimes	Usually	Always
Home Health Aide submits time slip and other paperwork in timely way	Seldom	Sometimes	Usually	Always

COMMENT SECTION

Please comment on the following and add your narrative below as a summary.

Record your impression of the employee' s willingness and cooperation.

Record your impression of the kind of relationship the employee maintains with clients/families.

Record your impression of the quality of work, follow-through and thoroughness of this employee's performance.

Record your impression of the clinical and technical understanding and care given by this Home Health Aide.

General summary:

Recommendations:

Areas for improvement:

Goals for next period:

Signature: ______________________________

Reviewer: ______________________________ Date: ________________

Employee: ______________________________ Date: ________________

Administrator: ______________________________ Date: ________________

Salary Change* approval: ______________________________ Date: ________________

Benefit Change* approval: ______________________________ Date: ________________

____

*Itemize changes below.

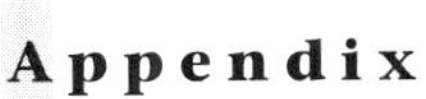
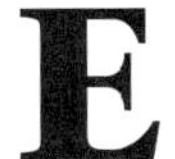

Appendix E

Reference Check Home Health Aide

Please complete and return to: ____

The following person ______________________________ has applied for employment with this company. Your name was given to us as a reference. All information is held confidentially. Please return your completed form to us as soon as possible.

Your name: ______________________________ Address: ______________________________

Position: ______________________________ Relationship to applicant: ______________________

How long you have known the applicant: ________________

Please rate applicant's skills according to the following scale, and circle answer:

1—Never 2—Sometimes 3—Most of the time 4—Always

1. Does applicant demonstrate good organizational skills? 1 2 3 4
   Comments:

2. Does applicant demonstrate efficient use of time? 1 2 3 4
   Comments:

3. Does applicant demonstrate common sense safety knowledge? 1 2 3 4
   Comments:

4. Does applicant demonstrate ability to be comfortable caring for infants and/or young children? 1 2 3 4
   Comments:

5. Do you feel the applicant is comfortable caring for adult clients recuperating from hospital stay, sickness or illness? 1 2 3 4
   Comments:

6. Does applicant demonstrate courtesy and respect for others? 1 2 3 4
   Comments:

7. Does applicant demonstrate reliability and punctuality? 1 2 3 4
   Comments:

8. Does applicant demonstrate good communication skills? 1 2 3 4
   Comments:

9. Does applicant demonstrate good basic knowledge of cooking skills? 1 2 3 4
   Comments:

Appendix F

Module 1: Safety

1. Should you always check the temperature of the bath water each time the child gets in?

   Yes _____ No _____

2. Should you ever leave a child unattended in the kitchen?

   Yes _____ No _____

3. Should you always have a baby in the same room with you, at all times?

   Yes _____ No _____

4. Is the Home Health Aide required to contact the Home Care Supervisor after any emergency?

   Yes _____ No _____

5. To reduce pain in minor burns, should you run cold water over the burn?

   Yes _____ No _____

6. If a child has a head injury, should you let them go right to sleep?

   Yes _____ No _____

7. Should you wash your hands before trying to touch any open wound?

   Yes _____ No _____

8. If a postpartum mother is experiencing excessive bleeding should you have her go straight to bed?

   Yes _____ No _____

9. In case of large fire, should you call the fire department after the entire house has been evacuated?

   Yes _____ No _____

Answers to Module I: Safety

1. yes
2. no
3. yes
4. yes
5. yes
6. no
7. yes
8. yes
9. yes

Module 2: Household Management

1. Is preparing meals, washing and folding clothes, dusting and other household chores part of the Home Health Aides duties?

   Yes _____ No _____

2. Should the Home Health Aide be organized in meal planning?

   Yes _____ No _____

3. Should the Aide check ingredients on food packages for any food allergies persons in the household may have?

   Yes _____ No _____

4. Should you review instructions prior to use of any electrical equipment?

   Yes _____ No _____

5. Should you ever mix any cleaning agents?

   Yes _____ No _____

6. Should you ever use bleach in household cleaning?

   Yes _____ No _____

7 List the components of household assessment.

8. Why do you do a family assessment?

Answers to Module II: Household Management

1. yes
2. yes
3. yes
4. yes
5. no
6. no
7. To provide a comfortable environment while meeting the client's daily needs for physical care and nutrition (instructor may find other acceptable answers).
8. To better know and understand the individual needs of the family (instructor may find similar answers acceptable).

Module 3: Infection Control

1. Is improper nutrition a factor in lowering the ability to fight off infection?

   Yes _____ No _____

2. Is an infection a germ causing illness?

   Yes _____ No _____

3. Can you pass an infection by touching someone's hand with germs on your hand?

   Yes _____ No _____

4. Should all Home Health Aides wash their hands as soon as they enter the household?

   Yes _____ No _____

5. Can you help prevent the spread of germs by washing your hands frequently?

   Yes _____ No _____

6. Should you wear your uniform to work?

   Yes _____ No _____

7. Can jewelry carry germs?

   Yes _____ No _____

8. Should the Aide always wear closed toe shoes?

   Yes _____ No _____

9. Should your hair be pulled back and secured, if longer than mid-length?

   Yes _____ No _____

Answers to Module III: Infection Control

1. yes
2. yes
3. yes
4. yes
5. yes
6. no
7. yes
8. yes
9. yes

Module 4: Communication

1. The home health aide can best begin to create an accepting atmosphere by being a good ___________ .

2. Communication may be putting feelings into words, or using facial expressions, posture, body tone, etc.

   Yes _____ No _____

3. "I hate being pregnant, I'm always tired and in pain, and I'm sick of being on bedrest." List one possible open response to your client's statements:

   List one possible closed response:

4. Indicate whether the following are positive communication techniques (P) or negative communication techniques (N).

   a. ________ using silence
   b. ________ giving information
   c. ________ giving approval
   d. ________ seeking clarification
   e. ________ interpreting
   f. ________ making observations

5. "I just can't cope with everything today. I'm tired." Which of the following would be the most appropriate response for the HHA:

   a. So, go to bed.
   b. Yes, you seem tired today.
   c. Come on, you can do it!
   d. Can we watch some TV now?

6. Your client begins to cry for no apparent reason. Which of the following would be the most appropriate response for the HHA?

   a. Why don't you go to the bedroom so you don't wake the baby?
   b. Oh, don't cry. It'll get better soon.
   c. I'm here. Would you like to talk?
   d. Walk away and leave the client alone.

7. Why is it important to watch for nonverbal communication, even when a client says he/she is feeling fine?

Answers to Communication test

1. listener

2. yes

3. Tell me more about the pain (the answer seeks a positive response).

   Well, go to bed (answer seeks to determine if HHA can identify negative response that should not occur).

4. a. p d. p
   b. p e. n
   c. n f. p

5. b

6. c

7. Demonstrates feelings, i.e., crying–sad, pacing–anxiety.

General Knowledge Test

1. What is the most important concern of the Home Health Aide?
2. Name two ways to develop a good relationship with child in your care?

   A. ____________________ B. ____________________
3. Is the sleep requirements the same for every child?

   Yes _____ No _____
4. Can you discipline with love and affection?

   Yes _____ No _____
5. Can signs of anxieties be shown with the arrival of a new authority figure in the household?

   Yes _____ No _____
6. To be strong and healthy, do children need good food, fresh air, and protection from danger?

   Yes _____ No _____
7. Are the physical and emotional needs of children the same everywhere?

   Yes _____ No _____
8. Will encouraging children to pick up after themselves, hang up their clothes, and having them help with the dishes promote better responsibility in the child?

   Yes _____ No _____
9. Should you praise acceptable behavior?

   Yes _____ No _____
10. Should you always check with the family for patterns of discipline for the child or make up your own?

    Check with family _____ Make up your own _____

Answers to General Knowledge Test

1. Provide safety for the needs of the client.
2. Develop trust, offer kindness (instructor may accept other answers; this is meant to demonstrate general attitude of aide towards child).
3. no
4. yes
5. yes
6. yes
7. no
8. yes
9. yes
10. Check with family.

Documentation Test

1. Documentation includes which of the following:
   a. HHA'S opinions about the client.
   b. Information about the weather.
   c. Information about the client's environment.

2. Documentation always includes which of the following:
   a. Client's temperature, pulse, respiration and blood pressure
   b. HHA's opinions on why a vital sign is abnormal.
   c. Only abnormal vital signs,
   d. Client's temperature, pulse and respiration.

Answer True or False to the following statements.

3. Any time a client is going against doctor's orders (e.g., ignoring bedrest orders), it should be documented. ________

4. Any change in a client's condition while the HHA is with the client should be documented. ________

5. Time of HHA arrival and departure from the client's home should be documented. ________

Answers to Documentation Test

1. c
2. a.
3. true
4. true
5. true

Home Health Aide Training

Supervised Practical

GOAL

Enable each student to become competent in recognizing and reporting emergencies.

OBJECTIVES

- To recognize and report emergencies to appropriate persons.
- To learn appropriate actions to take for client in emergency.

POLICY

Documentation of sixteen hours supervised laboratory and classroom experience prior to home health aide direct care of clients as ability to demonstrate performance practicum. Lecture and laboratory performance on clients will occur on and according to those items on pre-supervised training activity forms.

PROCEDURE

Instructor will document any comments and observations of satisfactory or unsatisfactory completion of activities directly on the Supervised Training Activities forms and place in personnel file of prospective employee.

(S)—satisfactory or (U)—unsatisfactory must be noted for each activity.

Time: ________ Activity: ________ Instructor's Signature: ______________________________

- demonstration of hot compress
- cold applications
- dressings and simple treatments
- obtaining weights
- ostomy care
- demonstration on dummy in maintaining and restoring breathing and foreign body in airway
- demonstrate actions for control of bleeding
- practice care for shock

Supervised Practical Training Activity

Home Health Aide Name: ______________________________ Date: ________

RN Instructor name: ______________________________

GOAL

Enable each student to become competent in taking vital signs

OBJECTIVES

1. Know how to take oral, axillar and rectal temperatures.
2. Know how to take wrist and apical pulse.
3. Know how to take BP.
4. Know how to assess respiration.
5. Know normal and abnormal values and quality.

SUPERVISION

Demonstrate and explain process

Allow students to take vital signs on other students

Home Health Aide Record of Vital Signs

Temperature ________ Pulse ________ Blood Pressure ________

Registered Nurse Qualified Instructor: ______________________________

Verification by RN of Home Health Aide Accuracy

Temperature ________ Pulse ________ Blood Pressure ________

Home Health Aide Practicum

Documentation of Supervised Practical Training—Home Health Aide Training Program. To be completed and maintained in personnel file.

Asterisks (*) indicate activities required for evaluation of the Aide's performance with client. Procedures performed on an individual client under the direction of a Qualified Registered Nurse Instructor and/or Evaluator are required for a license and certification.

Name: ______________________ Date: ______________

Where Observed: ______________ Degree of Competency: ______________

Final Disposition: ______________

Document supervised activity with Satisfactory (S) or Unsatisfactory (U).

KNOWLEDGE AND PRACTICAL SKILLS	IN FIELD	NOT OBS'D	IN CLASS
1. Recognizes signs/symptoms of illness.			
2. Reports and records signs/symptoms of illness according to agency procedures.			
*3. Takes temperature, pulse, respiration.			
4. Uses procedures that prevent the spread of infection when providing personal care.			
*5. Assists in personal hygiene, grooming, including:			
*a. bed bath (adult/child)			
*b. sponge, tub or shower bath			
*c. shampoo, sink, tub, or bed			
*d. nail and skin care			
*e. oral hygiene/feeding infant			
*f. toileting and elimination			
*6. Makes occupied beds, improvising when necessary.			
*7. Performs tasks using good body mechanics.			
*8. Demonstrates safe transfer techniques.			
*9. Assists person in ambulation.			
*10. Demonstrates normal range of motion.			
*11. Positions person in bed.			

Appendix G

Department of Health and Human Services
Health Care Financing Administration

Form Approved
OMB No. 0938-0357

HOME HEALTH CERTIFICATION AND PLAN OF TREATMENT

1. Patient's HI Claim No.	2. SOC Date	3. Certification Period From: To:	4. Medical Record No.	5. Provider No.

6. Patient's Name and Address	7. Provider's Name and Address

8. Date of Birth:
9. Sex ☐ M ☐ F
10. Medications: Dose/Frequency/Route (N)ew (C)hanged

11. ICD-9-CM	Principal Diagnosis	Date
12. ICD-9-CM	Surgical Procedure	Date
13. ICD-9-CM	Other Pertinent Diagnoses	Date

14. DME and Supplies
15. Safety Measures:
16. Nutritional Req.
17. Allergies:

18.A. Functional Limitations
1 ☐ Amputation
2 ☐ Bowel/Bladder (Incontinence)
3 ☐ Contracture
4 ☐ Hearing
5 ☐ Paralysis
6 ☐ Endurance
7 ☐ Ambulation
8 ☐ Speech
9 ☐ Legally Blind
A ☐ Dyspnea with Minimal Exertion
B ☐ Other (Specify)

18.B. Activities Permitted
1 ☐ Complete Bedrest
2 ☐ Bedrest BRP
3 ☐ Up as Tolerated
4 ☐ Transfer Bed/Chair
5 ☐ Exercises Prescribed
6 ☐ Partial Weight Bearing
7 ☐ Independent at Home
8 ☐ Crutches
9 ☐ Cane
A ☐ Wheelchair
B ☐ Walker
C ☐ No Restrictions
D ☐ Other (Specify)

19. Mental Status
1 ☐ Oriented
2 ☐ Comatose
3 ☐ Forgetful
4 ☐ Depressed
5 ☐ Disoriented
6 ☐ Lethargic
7 ☐ Agitated
8 ☐ Other

20. Prognosis
1 ☐ Poor
2 ☐ Guarded
3 ☐ Fair
4 ☐ Good
5 ☐ Excellent

21. Orders for Discipline and Treatments (Specify Amount/Frequency/Duration)

22. Goals/Rehabilitation Potential/Discharge Plans

23. Verbal Start of Care and Nurse's Signature and Date Where Applicable:

24. Physician's Name and Address

25. Date HHA received Signed POT

26. I ☐ certify ☐ recertify that the above home health services are required and are authorized by me with a written plan for treatment which will be periodically reviewed by me. This patient is under my care, is confined to his home, and is in need of intermittent skilled nursing care and/or physical or speech therapy or has been furnished home health services based on such a need and no longer has a need for such care or therapy, but continues to need occupational therapy.

27. Attending Physician's Signature (required on 485 Kept on File in Medical Records of HHA

Date Signed

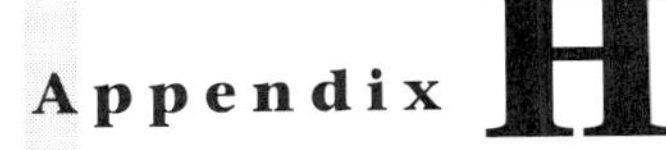

Consent for Treatment, Release of Information, Assignment of Benefits, Notice of Client Rights

Client Name: ____

Address: ____

City: ______________________ State: ________ Zip: ______________

I, ______________________, ______________ of ______________ intending to be
(custodial parent or legal guardian) (relationship) (minor client)

legally bound, hereby:

1. Consent to such care and treatment by ______________________, and its employees and agents (collectively, the "Agency"), as prescribed by the client's physician or dictated by the client's condition.
2. Authorize the Agency to release any medical records in its possession concerning the client as may be required by law or to pay benefits on the client's behalf. I authorize the client's physicians, insurers, and hospitals to release such medical records to the Agency at the Agency's request.
3. Authorize my insurer to disclose to the Agency the terms and extent of my coverage, and the amount of payments made to me for services provided by the Agency.
4. Assign, transfer, and set over to the Agency all of my or the client's rights to insurance proceeds or other funds to which I am or the client is or will become entitled as a result of the services rendered by the Agency.
5. Consent to and authorize payment, which would otherwise be payable to me or the client, to be made directly to the Agency. The Agency may issue a receipt for such payment which shall discharge the insurance company of its obligations under the policy to the extent of such payment.
6. Agree that I remain individually responsible to pay the Agency for all charges not paid for any reason by the insurer or other third-party payor. I understand that payment in full is due upon receipt of my bill. If payment for the Agency's services is made directly to me by my insurer, I agree to endorse the check to the Agency and forward it to the Agency within three days of receipt.

A photocopy of this document, if executed, shall be considered as effective and valid as the original.

The effect of this form and the Client's Rights and Responsibilities on the back of this form have been explained to me by the Agency and I understand its content and significance.

Date: ______________ Signature: ______________________

Name: ______________________
(please print)

Appendix I

Home Health Care Client's Bill of Rights/Responsibilities

As a home health care client you have the right to:

1. Standard: Right to be informed and to participate in planning care and treatment (1) The client has the right to be informed in advance about the care to be furnished.
2. Be given information about your rights and responsibilities for receiving home health care services, in terms and language you can reasonably expect to understand.
3. Receive a timely response from the Home Health Care Agency regarding your request for home health care services.
4. Be given information of the Home Health Care Agency charges and policy concerning payment for services, including your eligibility for third party reimbursement.
5. Choose your home health care providers.
6. Be given appropriate and professional quality home health care services without discrimination against your race, creed, color, religion, sex, national origin, sexual preference, handicap, or age.
7. The client's family or guardian may exercise the client's rights when the client has been judged incompetent.
8. The HHA must investigate complaints made by a client or the client's family or guardian regarding treatment or care that is (or fails to be) furnished, or regarding the lack of respect for the client's property by anyone furnishing services on behalf of the HHA, and must document both the existence of the complaint and the resolution of the complaint.
9. Be treated with courtesy and respect by all who provide home health care services to you; to have your property treated with respect.
10. Before the care is initiated, the HHA must inform the client, orally and in writing, of
    a. The extent of which payment may be expected from Medicare, Medicaid, or any other federally funded or aided program known to the HHA
    b. The charges for services that will not be covered by Medicare; and
    c. The charges that the individual may have to pay
    d. The client has the right to be advised orally and in writing of any changes in payment from last financial counseling.
11. The client has the right to be advised orally and in writing of any changes in payment. The HHA must advise the client of these changes orally and in writing as soon as possible, but no later than 15 working days from the date that the HHA becomes aware of a change.

12. Be given the necessary information so you will be able to give informed consent for your treatment prior to the start of any treatment.

13. Participate in the development of your home health care plan, to be informed in advance about the care to be provided and any changes in the care to be provided, including anticipated transfer of your care to another health care facility and/or termination of home health care service.

14. To be advised in advance of the disciplines that will provide care, and the frequency of visits proposed to be provided.

15. Be given data privacy and confidentiality; review your clinical record at your request.

16. Voice grievances regarding treatment or care that is (or fails to be) furnished, or regarding any lack of respect for privacy by anyone who is furnishing services on behalf of the home health care agency, without being subject to discrimination or reprisal for doing so.

    * Call ____________________ to voice a grievance and/or recommend changes in policies or services.
    * Medicare/Medicaid clients may also call a Hotline # (1-800-222-0989) to report grievances from 8:30 am–5:00 pm with answering service for non-business hours. This is *not* the number to reach the Home Health Care Agency or to obtain Medicare coverage/billing information.

17. Refuse all or part of your care to the extent permitted by law; to be informed of the expected consequences of such action.

18. The client's family or guardian may exercise the client's rights when the client has been judged incompetent.

Client Responsibilities

As a home health care client you have the responsibility to:

1. Give accurate and complete health information concerning your past illnesses, hospitalizations, medications, allergies, and other pertinent items.
2. Assist in developing and maintaining a safe environment.
3. Inform the Home Health Care Agency when you will not be able to keep a home health care visit.
4. Participate in the development and update of your home health care plan.
5. Adhere to your developed/updated home health care plan.
6. Request further information concerning anything you do not understand.
7. Give information regarding concerns and problems you have to Home Health Care Agency staff member.

Advance Directives

An advance directive is a written instruction, such as a living will or durable power of attorney for health care, recognized under state law, relating to the provision of health care when an individual's condition makes him/her unable to express his/her wishes. The intent of these provisions is to enhance an individual's control over medical treatment decisions.

The Agency's policy regarding implementation of a client's advance directive is to comply to the best of its ability with those instructions.

1. The client has been informed of the state living will law. Yes _____ No _____
2. Does the client have a living will? Yes _____ No _____
3. If so, is there a copy of the advance directive in the client's medical record? Yes _____ No _____

Client Signature: ______________________________ Date: ____________________

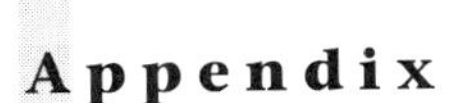
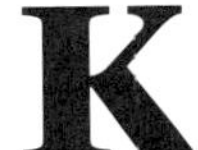

Appendix K

Initial Evaluation Form

Current Medical Profile

Client Name: ______________________ Date of Birth: ______________

Address: ______________________ Phone: (   ) ______________

Primary Physician: ______________________

Physician Address: ______________________ Phone: (   ) ______________

Primary Diagnosis: ______________________ Secondary Diagnosis: ______________

Allergies: ______________________ Functional Limitations: ______________

Client's Primary Caregiver: ______________________ Relationship: ______________

PHYSICAL ASSESSMENT		NORM.	ABNORM.	DESCRIBE/MEASURE/PAST MEDICAL HISTORY
SKIN	Color			
	Condition/Turgor			
METABOLIC	Temperature			
NEURO	Mental Status/ Headaches/Blackouts			
	Activity/Gait			
	Pupils			
	Seizures			
HEENT	Appearance			
	Neck Mobility			
	Lymph Nodes			
CARDIO-VASCULAR	Apical Pulse			
	Peripheral Pulse			
	Blood Pressure			
	Circulation/Capillary Refill			
CHEST	Configuration/Circumference			
	Auscultation			
	Respiration/Rate			
PSYCHO-SOCIAL	Interactions			
	Affect			
	Developmental Milestones			
MUSCULO/SKELETAL	Upper Extremities			
	Lower Extremities			
ABDOMEN	Shape			
	Bowel Sounds			
	Palpation			
GU	Voiding			
	BM			

RN Signature: ______________________ License #: ______________ Date: ________

Current Medical Profile

Client Name: ______________________

NUTRITIONAL STATUS	
	PO/Enteral
	Parenteral
	Feeding Issues weight

SAFETY ASSESSMENT	YES	NO	COMMENTS
Teaching Basic Home Safety			
CPR Training Reviewed/Reinforced			
Reviewed plan for emergency medical situation/emergency phone numbers			
Is do not resuscitate order applicable?			If yes, signed order must be in clinical record
Reviewed safety instruction related to equipment and care being provided			
Physical/Psychosocial Environment Adequate for Client Care			

Other medical personnel providing care (specify name and phone): ______________________

Insurance: ____________ ID#: ____________ Caseworker: ____________

Phone: ____________

If no insurance, why? ______________________

List equipment in home/specify instructions for use given: ______________________

____

Reason for Visit/Homecare Needs: ______________________

Nursing Diagnosis(es): ______________________

Short-Term Goal(s): ______________________

Long-Term Goal(s): ______________________

Nursing Interventions (treatment, teaching, etc.): ______________________

____

____

Evaluation (response to interventions): ______________________

____

____

____

Date and Nursing Care Plan for next visit: ______________________

____

Communication to M.D./Agency Office/Other: ______________________

Change in orders/Change in medication: ______________________

(Specify change and attach completed physician verbal order form)

RN Signature: ______________________ License #: ____________ Date: ________

Current Medication Profile

Client Name: ______________________________ Allergies: ______________________________

MEDICATION (Dose, Frequency, Rate)	MODIFICATION SINCE DATE OF REFERRAL	PURPOSE	SIGNIFICANT SIDE EFFECTS	INSTRUCTION *	UNDERSTANDING **
				____ ____ ____ ____ ____	____ ____ ____ ____ ____
				____ ____ ____ ____ ____	____ ____ ____ ____ ____
				____ ____ ____ ____ ____	____ ____ ____ ____ ____
				____ ____ ____ ____ ____	____ ____ ____ ____ ____
				____ ____ ____ ____ ____	____ ____ ____ ____ ____

Pharmacy: Phone:

* INSTRUCTION CODES:

1—Verbal Instructions given
2—Medication Sheet left in home
3—Medication Sheet & verbal instructions given
4—Side effects/adverse reactions reviewed
5—Dose & frequency reviewed
6—Purpose instructed
7—All of the above

** G—Good F—Fair P—Poor

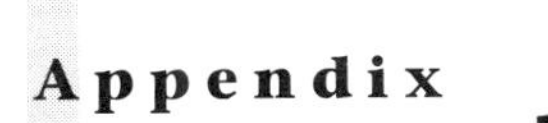
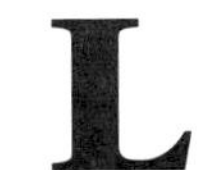

Appendix L

Pediatric Assessment and Care Screening for Function

To be completed by the nurse and used in developing the plan of care.

Section A. Identification and Background Information

1. ASSESSMENT DATE: ________________________________
2. CHILD'S NAME: ________________________________
3. SS#: ________________________________
4. MA./HMO I.D. #: ________________________________
5. REASON FOR ASSESSMENT
   ____ initial evaluation
   ____ hosp. reass.
   ____ readmission assessment
   ____ significant change in status
   ____ other
   ____ annual assessment
6. RESPONSIBILITY/LEGAL GUARDIAN
   ____ parent
   ____ legal guardian
7. ADVANCED DIRECTIVES
   ____ living will
   ____ organ donation
   ____ feeding restrictions
   ____ other treatment restrictions
   ____ none of the above
   ____ DNR ____ do not hosp.
   ____ autopsy request
   ____ med. restrictions
8. DISCHARGE PLANNED WITHIN 3 MONTHS
   ____ no ____ yes
   ____ unknown, uncertain
9. PARTICIPATE IN ASSESSMENT
   child: ____ yes ____ no
   family: ____ yes ____ no
   guardian: ____ yes ____ no

Section B. Cognitive Patterns

1. COMATOSE: ____ yes ____ no
2. CHANGE IN COGNITIVE STATUS: ____ yes ____ no
   Change in child's cognitive status, skills, or abilities in last 90 days:
   ___ no change ____ improved ____ deteriorated

Section C. Communication/Hearing Patterns

1. HEARING: ____ hears and turns to sound
   ____ does not respond to sound

2. COMMUNICATION DEVICES/TECHNIQUES
   ____ hearing aid, present and used
   ____ hearing aid, present and not used
   ____ other receptive Comm. techniques used, e.g., lip reading
   ____ none of the above

3. MAKING SELF UNDERSTOOD
   A. All Children
      ____ communicates what he/she wants
      ____ sometimes communicates what he/she wants
      ____ rarely/never communicates what he/she wants
   B. Children < 1 year old
      ____ smiles, coos, babbles or uses other sounds
      ____ sometimes smiles, coos, babbles or uses other sounds
      ____ rarely/never smiles, coos, babbles or uses other sounds
   C. Children 2 years or older
      ____ communicates with words so others can understand
      ____ sometimes communicates with words so others can understand
      ____ rarely/never communicates with words so others can understand
   D. Children over 3 years
      ____ understood
      ____ usually understood—difficulty finding words or finishing thoughts
      ____ sometimes understood—ability is limited to making concrete requests
      ____ rarely/never understood

4. CHANGE IN COMMUNICATION/HEARING
   ____ child's ability to express, understand or hear information has changed over last 90 days
   ____ no change ____ improved ____ deteriorated

Section D. Vision Patterns

1. VISION (ability to see in adequate light and with glasses if used)
   A. Children < 1 year old
      ____ seems to look at things & tries to get objects that are near but beyond reach
      ____ sometimes seems to look at things & tries to get objects that are near but beyond reach
      ____ rarely/never seems to look at things or tries to get objects that are near but beyond reach
   B. Children 2 years or older
      ____ adequate—sees fine detail, including regular print in books
      ____ impaired—sees large print, but not reg. print in books
      ____ highly impaired—limited vision; not able to see newspaper headlines; appears to follow objects with eyes
      ____ severely impaired—no vision or appears to see only light, colors, or shapes

2. VISUAL LIMITATIONS/DIFFICULTIES
   ____ side vision problems— decreased peripheral vision (e.g., leaves food on one side of tray, difficulty traveling, bumps into people and objects, misjudges placement of chair when seating self)
   ____ experiences any of following: sees halos or rings around lights; sees flashes of light; sees "curtains" over eyes
   ____ none of the above

3. VISUAL APPLIANCES
   ____ Glasses; contact lenses; lens implant, magnifying glass: ____ yes ____ no

Section E. Physical Functioning and Structural Problems

Section E. Physical Functioning and Structural Problems

1. ADL—all children 1 year or older
    ____ gets around the house without assistance
    ____ does things for him/herself that he/she should do
    ____ picks up and throws a ball or other object in intended direction
    ____ requires the same amount of help with eating as other children his/her age

2. ADL—all children 2 years or older
    ____ goes up and down stairs without assistance
    ____ participates in hard exercise or play
    ____ dresses him/herself
    ____ gets undressed without help

3. BODY CONTROL PROBLEMS
    ____ balance—partial or total loss of ability to balance self while standing
    ____ bedfast all or most of the time
    ____ contracture to arms, legs, shoulders, or hands
    ____ hemiplegia/hemiparesis—quadriplegia
    ____ arm—partial or total loss of voluntary movement
    ____ hand—lack of dexterity (e.g., problem using toothbrush or adjusting hearing aid)
    ____ leg—partial or total loss of voluntary movement
    ____ leg—unsteady gait
    ____ trunk—partial or total loss of ability to position, balance, or turn body
    ____ amputation
    ____ none of above

4. MOBILITY APPLIANCES/DEVICES
    ____ cane/walker
    ____ other person wheels
    ____ none of the above
    ____ brace/prosthesis
    ____ lifted (manually/mechanically)
    ____ wheels self

5. CHANGE IN ADL FUNCTION—change in ADL self-performance in last 90 days
    ____ no change ____ improved ____ deteriorated

Section F. Continence Self-Control Categories

Code for child performance:

0. Continent—complete control appropriate for age
1. Usually continent—bladder, incontinent episodes lx/wk or less; bowel, less than weekly
2. Occasionally incontinent—bladder 2+ times a week but not daily; bowel, once a week
3. Frequently incontinent—bladder, tended to be incontinent daily, but some control present: bladder 2+ times a week but not daily; bowel 2–3 times a week
4. Incontinent—had inadequate control, bladder, multiple daily episodes; bowel, all, or almost all, of the time

____ BOWEL CONTINENCE—control of bowel movement, with appliance of bowel continence programs, if employed

____ BLADDER CONTINENCE—control of urinary bladder function (if dribbles, volume insufficient to soak through underpants), with appliances (e.g., Foley) or continence programs, if employed

INCONTINENCE-RELATED TESTING (skip if child's bladder continence code equals 0 or 1 and no catheter is used)

____ child has been tested for a urinary tract infection
____ child has been checked for presence of a fecal impaction, or there is adequate bowel elimination
____ none of the above

APPLIANCES AND PROGRAMS

____ any scheduled toileting plan
____ external (condom) catheter
____ ostomy
____ peds/briefs used
____ enemas/irrigation
____ did not use toilet room/ commode/urinal
____ indwelling catheter
____ intermittent catheter
____ none of above

CHANGE IN URINARY CONTINENCE

____ no change ____ improved ____ deteriorated

Section G. Psychosocial Well Being

1. SENSE OF INITIATIVE/INVOLVEMENT
   ____ at ease interacting with others
   ____ plays with other children
   ____ responds to attention

2. UNSETTLED RELATIONSHIPS
   ____ acts timid or shy
   ____ acts afraid of new situations
   ____ fights a lot with other children

Section H. Mood and Behavior Patterns

1. SAD OR ANXIOUS BEHAVIOR
   Demonstrated signs of mental distress
   ____ acts moody
   ____ seems unusually irritable or cross
   ____ seems unusually difficulty
   ____ has frequent temper tantrums
   ____ seems to feel sick and tired
   ____ reacts to little things by crying
   ____ acts restless and fidgety

2. MOOD PERSISTENCE
   ____ sad or anxious mood intrudes daily over last 7 days
   ____ not easily altered, doesn't "cheer up" ____ yes ____ no

3. PROBLEM BEHAVIOR
   Code for behavior in last 7 days:
   0. Behavior not exhibited in last 7 days
   1. Behavior of this type occurred less than daily
   2. Behavior of this type occurred daily or more frequently

____ WANDERING (moved with no rational purpose, seemingly oblivious to needs or safety)
____ VERBALLY ABUSIVE (others were threatened, screamed at, cursed at)
____ PHYSICALLY ABUSIVE (others were hit, shoved, scratched, sexually abused)
____ SOCIALLY INAPPROPRIATE/DISRUPTIVE BEHAVIOR (made disrupting sounds, noisy, screams, self-abusive acts, sexual behavior or disrobing in public, smeared/threw food/feces)

4. CHILD RESISTS CARE (check all types of resistance that occurred in the last 7 days)
   ____ resisted taking medications/injection
   ____ resisted ADL assistance
   ____ none of the above

5. BEHAVIOR MANAGEMENT PROGRAM (Behavior problem has been addressed by clinically developed behavior management program. (*Note:* Do not include programs that involve only physical restraints or psychotropic medications in this category.)
   0. No behavior problem 1. Yes, addressed 2. No, not addressed

6. CHANGE IN MOOD (in last 90 days)
   0. No change 1. Improved 2. Deteriorated

7. CHANGE IN PROBLEM BEHAVIOR
   0. No change 1. Improved 2. Deteriorated

Section I. Activity Pursuit Patterns

1. SLEEP PATTERNS—All Children
   ____ sleeps well/through the night (if appropriate for age)
   ____ nap time and frequency appropriate for age

   Children 2 years or older
   a. During the past 2 wks did child spend all or part of the day in bed?
      ____ yes ____ no
   b. How many days did he/she stay in bed in the last 2 wks?

2. ACTIVITY—Children 1 year or older
   ____ concentrated or paid attention for a period of time
   ____ got involved in games or other play

3. ACTIVITY—Children 2 years or older
   ____ played games by him/herself

Section J. Disease Diagnoses

1. CURRENT ICD-9 CODES AND DIAGNOSES

   ________ ____
   ________ ____
   ________ ____
   ________ ____
   ________ ____

Section K. Health Conditions

1. PROBLEM CONDITIONS (check all that are present in last 7 days unless other time frame indicated)
   ____ constipation
   ____ dizziness/vertigo
   ____ fecal Impaction
   ____ hallucinations/delusions
   ____ joint pain
   ____ fainting
   ____ pain, daily or almost daily
   ____ none of above
   ____ diarrhea
   ____ edema
   ____ fever
   ____ internal bleeding
   ____ vomiting
   ____ shortness of breath
   ____ recurrent lung aspirations in last 90 days

2. HOSPITALIZATIONS
   ____ hospitalized in past 30 days
   ____ hospitalized in past 31–180 days
   ____ number of days hospitalized

3. STABILITY OF CONDITIONS
   ____ conditions/diseases make child's cognitive, ADL, or behavior status unstable—fluctuating, precarious, or deteriorating
   ____ child experiencing an acute episode or a flare-up of a recurrent/chronic problem
   ____ none of the above

Section L. Oral/Nutritional Status

1. ORAL PROBLEMS
   ____ chewing problem
   ____ mouth pain
   ____ swallowing problem
   ____ none of the above

2. HEIGHT AND WEIGHT
   ____ height ____ weight

   Weight loss (i.e., 5% in last 30 days; or 10% in last 180 days)
   ____ yes ____ no

3. NUTRITIONAL PROBLEMS
   ____ complaints about the taste of many foods
   ____ insufficient fluid: dehydrated
   ____ did NOT consume all/almost all liquids provided during last 3 days
   ____ regular complaint of hunger
   ____ leaves 25%+ food uneaten at most meals
   ____ none of the above

4. NUTRITIONAL APPROACHES
   ____ parenteral/IV
   ____ mechanically altered diet
   ____ therapeutic diet
   ____ none of the above
   ____ feeding tube
   ____ syringe (oral feeding)
   ____ dietary supplement between meals
   ____ plague guard, stab. built-up utensil, etc.

Section M. Oral/Dental Status

1. ORAL STATUS AND DISEASE PREVENTION
   ____ debris (soft, easily movable substances) present in mouth prior to going to bed at night
   ____ thrush
   ____ broken loose, or carious teeth
   ____ inflamed gums (gingiva); swollen or bleeding gums; oral abscesses, ulcers or rashes
   ____ daily cleaning of teeth/dentures
   ____ none of the above

Section N. Skin Condition

1. STASIS ULCER (open lesion caused by poor venous circulate to lower extremities): ____ yes ____ no

2. PRESSURE ULCERS
   Code for highest stage of pressure ulcer:
   0. No pressure ulcers
   1. Stage I: A persistent area of skin redness (w/out a break in the skin) that does not disappear when pressure is relieved
   2. Stage 2: A partial thickness loss of skin layers that presents clinically as an abrasion, blister, or shallow crater
   3. Stage 3: A full thickness of skin is lost, exposing the subcutaneous tissues—presents as a deep crater with or w/out undermining adjacent tissue
   4. Stage 4: A full thickness of skin and subcutaneous tissue is lost, exposing muscle and/or bone

3. HISTORY OF RESOLVED/CURED PRESSURE ULCERS
   Child has had a pressure ulcer that was resolved/cured in last 90 days. ____ yes ____ no

4. SKIN PROBLEMS/CARE
   ____ open lesions other than status or pressure ulcers (e.g., cuts)
   ____ skin desensitized to pain, pressure, discomfort
   ____ protective/preventive skin care
   ____ turning/repositioning program
   ____ pressure relieving beds, bed/chair pads (e.g., egg crate pads)
   ____ wound care/treatment (e.g., pressure ulcer care, surgical wound)
   ____ other skin care/treatment
   ____ none of the above

Section O. Medication Use

1. NUMBER OF MEDICATIONS (record # different meds used in last # days: enter 0 if none). ________

2. NEW MEDICATIONS (has child received any during the last 90 days?). ____ yes ____ no

3. INJECTIONS (record # days of injections of any type received during the last # days). ________
4. DAYS RECEIVED THE FOLLOWING MEDS (record # days during last # days; enter 0 if not used; 1 if long-acting meds, used less than weekly).
   ____ antipsychotics ____ antianxiety/hypnotics ____ antidepressants

5. Previous Med Results (skip this question if child currently receiving antipsychotics, antianxiety/hypnotics, or antidepressants:

   Child has previously received psychoactive medications for a mood or behavior problem, and these medications were effective (without undue adverse consequences)
   0. No, drugs not used
   1. Drugs were effective
   2. Drugs were not effective
   3. Drug effectiveness unknown

Section P. Special Treatment and Procedures

1. SPECIAL TREATMENTS AND PROCEDURES
   Special Care—check treatments received during the last 14 days
   ____ chemotherapy ____ radiation ____ dialysis
   ____ suctioning ____ trach care ____ IV meds
   ____ transfusions ____ 0_2 ______________ other
   ____ none of the above

   Therapies—record the # of days each of the following therapies was administered (for at least 10 minutes during a day) in the last 7 days.
   ____ speech—language pathology and audiology services
   ____ OT ____ PT—psychological therapy (any licensed prof) ____ RT

2. ABNORMAL LAB VALUES
   Has child had any abnormal lab values during the last 90 days?
   ____ yes ____ no ____ no tests performed

3. DEVICES AND RESTRAINT
   ____ 0. not used ____ 1. used less than daily ____ 2. used daily
   ____ bed rail ____ trunk restraint ____ limb restraint ____ chair prevents rising

Background Information Intake at Admission

I. IDENTIFICATION INFORMATION

1. RESIDENT NAME: ____
   First Last

2. DATE OF CURRENT ADMISSION: ________________

3. TYPE OF INS.: ________________ INS. NO.: ________________

4. FACILITY PROVIDER #: ________________

5. GENDER: ________________ 6. RACE: ________________

7. DOB: ________________ 8. PRIMARY LANGUAGE: ________________

9. MENTAL HEALTH HISTORY
   Does child's record indicate any history of MH/MR, or any other mental health problem?
   ____ yes ____ no

10. CONDITIONS RELATED TO MR/MH STATUS (check all conditions that were manifested before age 22 and are likely to continue indefinitely)

    ____ Not applicable—no MR/Do (skip to item 11)

    MR/Do with organic condition
    ____ CP ____ Down's syndrome ____ autism ____ epilepsy

    Other organic condition related to MR/Do
    ____ MR/Do with no organic condition ____ Unknown

11. ADMITTED FROM: ____ private home or apt. ____ hospital ____ other

12. ADMISSION INFORMATION AMENDED (check all that apply)
    ____ accurate information unavailable
    ____ observation revealed additional information
    ____ child unstable at admission

II. BACKGROUND INFORMATION AT RETURN/READMISSION

1. Date of current readmission: ____________________
2. Admission Information amended (check all that apply)
   ____ accurate information unavailable earlier
   ____ observation revealed additional information
   ____ resident unstable at admission

RN Signature: ____ Date: ____________________

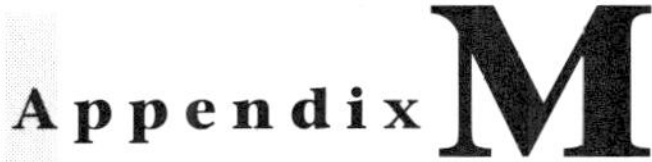

Nursing Plan of Care and Progress Record

HHA Supervisory Visit	Yes ____	No ____	
PT satisfied with care?	Yes ____	No ____	
HHA Following Care Plan	Yes ____	No ____	
Care plan updated?	Yes ____	No ____	
HHA's name ______________________			

CLIENT NAME: ______________________

ADDRESS: ______________________

____

____

PHONE: (   ) ______________________

ALLERGIES: ______________________

LEAD SCREENING STATUS
1. Is infant the appropriate age for lead screening? Yes ____ No ____
2. If yes, does caregiver know if it was done? Yes ____ No ____
3. Does caregiver know results? Yes ____ No ____

IMMUNIZATION STATUS
1. Did infant receive any immunizations at last visit? Yes ____ No ____
2. Has infant received any immunizations since birth? Yes ____ No ____
3. If yes, when and which ones? (if changed from last visit): ______________________
   Name of last pediatric provider: ______________________
4. Is infant appropriately immunized (as reported by caregiver)? Yes ____ No ____
5. If no, why? (as explained by caregiver): ______________________

Date of last appt.: ________ Date of next appt.: ________

SKILLED OBSERVATION/ASSESSMENT

	Normal	Abnormal	Describe		Normal	Abnormal	Describe
Metabolic (TPR)				Genitourinary			
HEENT				Musculoskeletal			
Cardiovascular				Neurological			
Respiratory				Integumentary			
ABD/G.I.				Psychosocial			
Nutrition/Wt.				Other			

Medical Diagnosis: ______________________

Reason for Visit/Homecare Needs: ______________________

Nursing Diagnosis(es): ______________________

Short-Term Goal(s): ______________________

Long-Term Goal(s): ______________________

Nursing Interventions (treatment, teaching, etc.): ______________________

____

____

Evaluation (response to interventions): ______________________

____

____

Date and Nursing Care Plan for next visit: ______________________

____

Communication to M.D./Agency Office/Other: ______________________

Changes in orders/changes in medication: ______________________

(specify change and attach completed verbal order form)

RN Signature: ______________________ License #: ______________ Date: __________

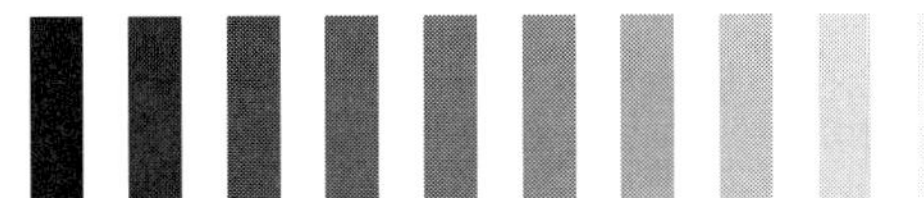

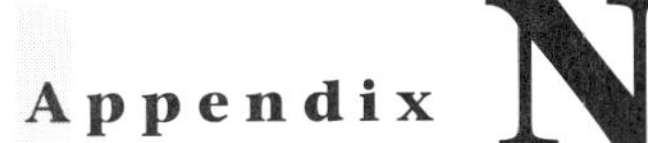

Appendix N

Supervisory Visit Note

Client Name: ______________________

Client Vital signs:
P ________ BP ________
R ________ T ________
(if indicated)

Employee supervised: ______________________

Employee discipline: ____ RN ____ HHA
____ LPN ____ Other

Assessment: Client's condition R/T employee's services: ______________________

____

____

Employee's performance R/T care plan: ______________________

____

____

Employee: ____ present ____ not present

Employee is: ____ punctual ____ properly dressed/groomed ____ considerate ____ thorough

Client's/family's comments: ______________________

____

____

____ Care plan reviewed/revised ____ On-the-job education provided

Supervisor's comments: ______________________

____

____

Supervisor's signature: ______________________ Date: ____________

cc: Employee File

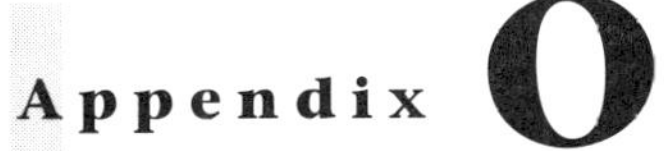

Appendix O

Home Health Aide Care Plan

Client Name: ______________________ D.O.B.: __________ Phone: __________
Address: ____
Date Start:: __________ Hrs/Day: __________ Days/Week: __________

TASK **INSTRUCTIONS**

VITAL SIGNS
___ Pulse ______________________
___ Resp. ______________________
___ BP ______________________
___ Temp ______________________
___ Weight ______________________
___ Precautions ______________________
____

HYGIENE ______________________
___ Bath ______________________
___ Perineal ______________________
___ Skin Care ______________________
___ Oral Care ______________________
___ Shampoo ______________________
___ Dressing assistance ______________________
___ Precautions ______________________
___ Other ______________________
____

ACTIVITY ______________________
___ Ambulation ______________________
___ Chair/wheelchair ______________________
___ Transfers ______________________
___ Reposition in bed ______________________
___ Range of motion ______________________
___ Precautions ______________________
___ Other ______________________
____

ELIMINATION
___ Assist to BSC/toilet ______________________
___ Bedpan ______________________
___ Catheter care ______________________
___ Incontinence care ______________________
___ Ostomy care ______________________
___ Record intake/output ______________________
___ Precautions ______________________
___ Other

TASK **INSTRUCTIONS**

NUTRITION
___ Meal Planning ______________________
___ Meal Preparations
Diet ______________________
Breakfast ______________________
Lunch ______________________
Dinner ______________________
Snacks ______________________
___ Fluids
Encourage ______________________
Restrict ______________________
___ Food
Restrictions ______________________
___ Precautions ______________________
___ Other ______________________

HOME MANAGEMENT
___ Kit/Bath/Liv/Bedroom ______________________
___ Linen change ______________________
___ Laundry
___ Childcare ______________________
____
____
____
___ Grocery Shopping/errands ______________________
___ Transport client ______________________
___ Other ______________________

MEDICATIONS
___ Notify office if ______________________
____
____
___ Other ______________________
____

EMERGENCY CONTACT: ______________________ PHONE: __________

SAFETY PRECAUTIONS

Client Caregiver
___ ___ ______________________
___ ___ ______________________
___ ___ ______________________

CARE PLAN REVIEW/CHANGES IN POT

Date By
____
____
____

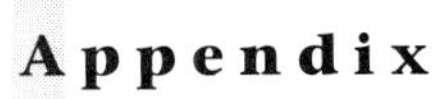
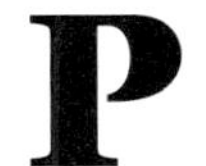

Appendix P

Home Health Aide Clinical Record

Client Name: ______________________ Shift Hours: ______________________
Home Health Aide Signature: ______________________ Nurse Supervisor: ______________________
CALL CLINICAL SUPERVISOR REGARDING CHANGE IN CARE OR CONDITION OF PATIENT

	M	T	W	TH	F	S	S
Enter date of visit							
Enter time in - out							
VITAL SIGNS: Record TPR under day obtained: Temp							
Pulse							
Resp.							
HYGIENE:							
Bath: Bed Tub/Shower							
Perineal							
Skin Care							
Oral Care							
Dressing assistance							
Other							
ACTIVITY:							
Bedrest positioning							
Transfer to bed/chair/wheelchair							
Ambulation with assistance/cane, crutches							
Exercises: range of motion							
Assistance with home PT/ST/OT program							
Other							
NUTRITION:							
Meal Planning/Preparation							
Feeding							
Encourage fluids							
Restrict fluids							
HOME MANAGEMENT:							
Kitchen/bathroom/living room/bedroom							
Linen change							
Laundry							
Childcare							
Grocery shopping/errands							
Transport client							
MEDICATIONS:							
Reminder							
Supervise/assist							
OTHER:							

NOTE: ____

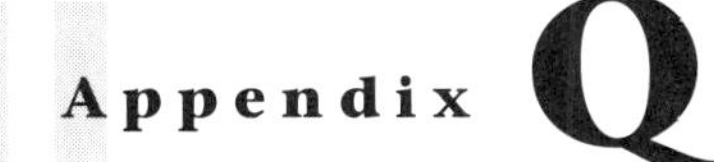

Appendix Q

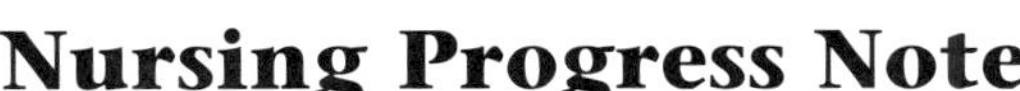

Nursing Progress Note

Client Name: ____________________

DATE	

Homemaker's Progress Note

CLIENT NAME: ______________________

DATE	

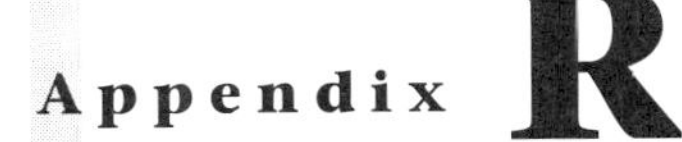

Appendix R

Pediatric Intake and Output Record for Parents' Use

Client Name: ______________________________

	Date/Day	Feeding Amt & Time	Amt & Time	Amt & Time	Amt & Time	Amt & Time	Amt & Time	Amt & Time	Total # of Feedings/ per day	Wet Diapers (Mark with X for each change)	Total # of wet diapers/day (void/cc)	BM
MONDAY												
TUESDAY												
WEDNESDAY												
THURSDAY												
FRIDAY												
SATURDAY												
SUNDAY												
MONDAY												
TUESDAY												
WEDNESDAY												
THURSDAY												
FRIDAY												
SATURDAY												
SUNDAY												

Appendix 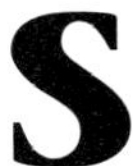

Discharge Summary

Insurance Co.: ____________________ ID#: ____________________

Client name: ____________________ Date of birth: ____________________

Address: ____________________

Diagnosis: ____________________

Date of first visit: __________ Date of last visit: __________

No. of visits: RN: ______ LPN: ______ PT: ______ OT: ______ ST: ______ HHA: ______ Other: __________ (type of service)

Date of discharge: __________

Initiation of discharge: Physician (give name): ____________________

Physician's address: ____________________

Agency: __________ Client/family: __________

Reason for termination of service: ____________________

____

SUMMARY OF PROGRESS AND CLIENT/PATIENT STATUS AT DISCHARGE (PHYSICAL, MENTAL, EMOTIONAL):

Subjective: ____________________

____

____

Objective: ____________________

____

Assessment: ____________________

____

____

		Attained	
GOALS:	____________________	Yes: ______	No: ______
	____________________	Yes: ______	No: ______
	____________________	Yes: ______	No: ______

PLAN:

Referrals made and final disposition: ____________________

____

____

Client/patient notified of discharge: Yes: ______ No: ______ Family notified of discharge: Yes: ______ No: ______

Physician notified of discharge: Yes: ______ No: ______

Signature: ____________________ Date: __________

Appendix **T**

Basic Policies and Procedures

POLICY: Vital signs will be taken as part of physical assessment.

PURPOSE:

- To count the number of times the client's heart beats per minute.
- To obtain an estimate of the quality of client's heart action.

PROCEDURE:

Radial Pulse:

1. Wash hands.
2. Support the arm along side the client with the wrist extended and the palm of the hand downward.
3. Place the first and second fingers along the radial artery and press gently against the radius. Rest the thumb in opposition to the fingers on the back of the client's wrist. Apply only enough pressure to feel the pulsating artery.

   Note rhythm, rate, and volume for 30 seconds. If irregularity is noted, take the pulse for one full minute.
4. Record pulse rate on proper assessment/clinical record form.

Apical Pulse:*

1. Wash hands.
2. Warm the stethoscope's diaphragm in your hand.
3. Place diaphragm of stethoscope over the point of maximum impulse, which is just lateral to the base of the left nipple.
4. Count the sound of each heartbeat, heard as "lub-dub," as one heartbeat.
5. Note rate for 30 seconds. If irregularity is noted, take apical rate for one full minute.
6. Record apical rate on proper assessment/clinical record form.

*An apical rate is taken on all children under two years of age and all those with cardiac problems, and/or upon physician's order.

POLICY: A respiratory rate assessment is taken on all clients, as indicated.

PURPOSE:

- To assess client's respiratory status.
- To assess client's respiratory rate.

PROCEDURE:

1. Wash hands.
2. Count infant, child's or adult's breathing rate for 30 seconds. If irregularity is noted, take rate for one full minute.
3. For infant (or child), place hand over infant's back or chest.
4. For adult, observe rise and fall of client's chest with each inspiration and expiration.
5. Assess the depth and character of respirations, client's skin color, and muscles used in breathing.
6. Record respiratory rate on proper assessment/clinical record form.

POLICY: Temperatures are taken on clients as appropriate.

PURPOSE: To measure client's body temperature.

PROCEDURE:

1. Wash hands.
2. Clean thermometer with an alcohol swab. Rinse it with cold water and dry thermometer.
3. Shake thermometer down to 96 degrees.
4. Axillary: For newborns, premature infants, and older children in whom oral temperatures are not feasible
   a. Wash hands
   b. Clean thermometer with an alcohol swab. Rinse it with cold water and then dry thermometer.
   c. Shake thermometer down to 96 degrees.

5. Oral: For older children or adults who are able to safely hold thermometer in mouth. Refrain from taking oral temperature on any client who is unconscious, exhibits irrational mouth breathing, or has disease of oral cavity.
   a. Wash hands.
   b. Clean thermometer with an alcohol swab. Rinse it with cold water and then dry thermometer.
   c. Shake thermometer down to 96 degrees.

   Patient is to hold thermometer under tongue for 3–5 minutes.

6. Rectal: For most children under 4 years old who do not have diarrhea, thrombocytopenia, or leukopenia, or who have not had rectal or perineal surgery.
   a. Wash hands.
   b. Clean thermometer with an alcohol swab. Rinse it with cold water and then dry thermometer.
   c. Shake thermometer down to 96 degrees.
   d. Put on disposable gloves.
   e. Position child either prone or lying on side; infant may be supine with knees flexed and feet held up.
   f. Lubricate thermometer with water-soluble lubricant.
   g. Insert bulb of thermometer into rectum $1/4$–$1/2$" and hold for 3 minutes.
   h. Record on proper assessment/clinical record form.

POLICY: Blood pressures are taken for all clients as indicated.

PURPOSE: To measure client's systolic and diastolic blood pressure by an indirect method.

PROCEDURE: Determining bladder and cuff size:

A. The inflatable bladder is surrounded by an unyielding covering, the cuff. The bladder must be the correct width for the diameter of the patient's arm. If it is too narrow, the blood pressure reading will be erroneously high; if it is too wide, the reading may be erroneously low. The proper cuff and bladder dimension combination is based on arm circumference, not the age of the patient or the cuff name. (See table below.)
B. Remove or roll up any clothing on the arm. Measure the upper arm circumference at the midpoint (half the distance from the acromion to the blecranon).
C. The bladder width should be 40% of the limb circumference. The bladder length should cover 60–100% of the limb circumference.
D. Ultrasonic methods: wider cuff bladders are more accurate. The width should be no less than 50% of the limb circumference.
E. Cuff size for the calf and thigh:
   1. Calf: Cuff size will be approximately the same as that for the arm.
   2. Thigh: Cuff size should be proportionately wider and longer than that for the arm.

Recommended Bladder Dimensions for Blood Pressure Cuff

Arm Circumference at Midpoint (cm)	*Cuff Name*	*Bladder Width (cm)*	*Bladder Length (cm)*
5–7.5	Newborn	3	5
7.5–13	Infant	5	8
13–20	Child	8	13
17–26	Small adult	11	17
24–32	Adult	13	24
32–42	Large adult	17	32
42–50	Thigh	20	42

PROCEDURE:

A. Measurement in the arm
1. Assist client to a comfortable position with the forearm supported and the palm of the hand upward.
2. Securely place the cuff around the upper arm so that the bladder of the cuff is midline over the brachial artery, and the lower edge of the blood pressure cuff is 2 cm above the antecubital fossa.
3. The pressure should be measured when the arm is at heart level. Place infants and children in supine position; older children and adults may be allowed to sit upright.
4. Palpate the radial artery. Inflate the cuff to approximately 39 mm Hg above the point where the radial pulse disappears.
5. Place the diaphragm of the stethoscope over the brachial artery and release the pressure at 2–3 mm Hg/second.
   a. The systolic pressure is the point when the initial tapping sound is heard. At least two connective beats should be heard as the pressure falls.
   b. The onset of muffling is the best index of diastolic pressure in children.
   c. The point when sounds become inaudible may be far below the intra-arterial diastolic pressure in infants and children.
6. When all sounds have disappeared, the cuff should be deflated rapidly and completely. One to two minutes should elapse before further determinations are made to allow release of blood trapped in veins.
7. Document reading on appropriate assessment or clinical record form. Notify physician of any significant changes in blood pressure reading.

B. Measurement in the Thigh
1. The child should lie face down and the cuff applied with the bladder over the posterior aspect of the mid-thigh.

   If the child is unable to lie face down, obtain the pressure reading with the child supine, by flexing the knee just enough to permit application of the stethoscope over the popliteal space.
2. Place the stethoscope over the popliteal fossa to obtain the reading.
3. The larger bladder usually records systolic pressure in the thigh as 10–40 mm Hg higher than that in the arm, but the diastolic pressure is essentially the same for both.

C. Measurement in the calf:
1. Position the distal border of the cuff at the malleoli.
2. Auscultate over the posterior tibial or dorsalis pedis artery.

D. Palpatory pressure
1. Inflate the cuff to approximately 200 mm Hg.
2. The reading is taken when the pulse distal to the cuff becomes palpable in the course of deflation.
3. This reading lies between the systolic and diastolic pressures obtained by the auscultatory method.

Common Abbreviations in Maternal–Child Nursing

ABC	alternative birthing center; airway, breathing, circulation
AC	abdominal circumference
ADA	American Diabetes Association
ADL	activities of daily living
AFP	alpha-fetoprotein
AFV	amniotic fluid volume
AGA	average for gestational age
AIDS	acquired immune deficiency syndrome
AROM	artificial rupture of membranes
BAT	brown adipose tissue (brown fat)
BGS	blood glucose sample
BL	baseline (fetal heart rate baseline)
BMR	basal metabolic rate
BOW	bag of waters
BP	blood pressure
BPD	biparietal diameter; bronchopulmonary dysplasia
BPM	beats per minute
BSE	breast self-examination
BUN	blood urea nitrogen
CC	chest circumference; cord compression; chief complaint
cc	cubic centimeter
CDC	Centers for Disease Control
CHF	congestive heart failure
CID	cytomegalic inclusion disease
CMV	cytomegalovirus
cm	centimeter
CNM	certified nurse-midwife
CNS	central nervous system
CPAP	continuous positive airway pressure
CPD	cephalopelvic disproportion; citrate–phosphate–dextrose
CPR	cardiopulmonary resuscitation
C/S	cesarean section or c-section
DHS	Department of Health Services
dil	dilatation
D&C	dilatation and curettage
DES	diethylstilbestrol
DFMR	daily fetal movement response
DM	diabetes mellitus
DOB	date of birth
DRG	diagnostic related groups

DTR	deep tendon reflexes
ECMO	extracorporeal membrane oxygenator
EDC	estimated date or confinement
EFA	essential fatty acid
EFM	electronic fetal monitoring
EFW	estimated fetal weight
EPIS	episiotomy
FAD	fetal activity diary
FAS	fetal alcohol syndrome
FBS	fetal blood sample; fasting blood sugar
FBM	fetal breathing movements
FHR	fetal heart rate
FHT	fetal heart tones
FM	fetal movement
FMD	fetal movement diary
FMR	fetal movement record
FPG	fasting plasma glucose
GDM	gestational diabetes mellitus
GI	gastrointestinal
GRAV	gravida
GTT	glucose tolerance test
GYN	gynecology
HCG	human chorionic gonadotrophin
HEENT	head, ears, eyes, nose, throat
HIV	human immunodeficiency virus
IDDM	insulin-dependent diabetes mellitus
IGT	impaired glucose tolerance
ITP	idiopathis thrombocytopenic purpura
IUFD	intrauterine fetal demise
IUGR	intrauterine growth retardation
IV	intravenous
JCAHO	Joint Commission for the Accreditation of Healthcare Organizations
L/S ratio	lecithin/sphingomyelin ratio
MAP	mean arterial pressure
NIDDM	non–insulin-dependent diabetes mellitus
NPO	nulla per os
NSCT	nipple stimulation challenge test
NST	non-stress test
OB	obstetric
OCT	oxytocin challenge test
PIH	pregancy-induced hypertension
PO	per os (by mouth)
PROM	premature rupture of membranes
RBC	red blood cell
RDS	Respiratory distress syndrome
RMA	right mentoanterior
ROA	right occiput anterior
ROM	rupture of membranes
ROP	right occiput posterior
ROP	retinopathy of prematurity
ROT	right occiput transverse
RMP	right mentoposterior
RMT	right mentotransverse
RSA	right sacroanterior
RSP	right sacroposterior

SFD	small for dates
SGA	small for gestational age
SIDS	sudden infant death syndrome
SOAP	subjective data, objective data, analysis, plan
SOB	short of breath
SROM	spontaneous rupture of the membranes
STD	sexually transmitted disease
TORCH	toxoplasmosis, other (viruses) rubella, cytomegalovirus, herpes virus type 2
TPN	total parenteral nutrition
TSS	toxic shock syndrome
U/A	urinalysis
UAC	umbilical artery catheter
UC	uterine contraction
UPI	uteroplacental insufficiency
UTI	urinary tract infection
VBAC	vaginal birth after cesarean
WBC	white blood cell
WIC	supplemental food program for woman, infants, and children
WNL	within normal limits

Glossary

abortion loss of pregnancy before the fetus is viable outside the uterus; miscarriage, or elective termination

abruptio placentae partial or total premature separation of a normally implanted placenta.

acceleration increase in the baseline fetal heart

acme peak; time of greatest intensity (of a uterine contraction)

acrocyanosis cyanosis of the extremities

afterbirth placenta and membranes expelled or "delivered" after the infant; referred to as the third stage of labor

afterbirth pains cramplike pains due to contractions of the uterus after childbirth

albinism a congenital absence of normal skin pigmentation

albuminuria readily detectable amounts of albumin in the urine

amenorrhea suppression or absence of menstruation

amniocentesis removal of amniotic fluid by insertion of needle into the amniotic sac (amniotic fluid is used to assess health and maturity status of fetus)

amnion the inner of the two uterine membranes that form the sac containing the fetus and the amniotic fluid

amniotic fluid the fluid surrounding the fetus in utero

amnionitis infection within the amniotic fluid

amniotomy the artificial rupturing of the amniotic sac

analgesic drug that relieves pain

anencephaly congenital deformity in which the cerebrum, cerebellum, and flat bones of the skull are absent

anesthesia partial or complete loss of sensation with or without loss of consciousness; excess amount of carbon dioxide in the body

anomaly a malformation; an organ or structure

anoxia deficiency of oxygen

antepartum time between conception and the onset of labor

anterior pertaining to the front

Apgar score a scoring system used to evaluate newborns at 1 minute and 5 minutes after delivery. The total score is derived by assessing five signs: heart rate, respiratory effort, muscle tone, reflex irritability, and color

apnea a condition that occurs when respirations cease for more than 20 seconds, with cyanosis

areola darker pigmented skin surrounding the nipple of the breast

Bartholin's glands	two small mucus glands on each side of the vaginal orifice that secrete small amounts of mucus during intercourse
bilirubin	orange or yellowish pigment in bile; a breakdown product of red blood cells that is carried by the blood to the liver, where it is excreted in the bile and in the stools.
brown adipose tissue	fat deposits in neonates that provide greater heat protection
caudal block	regional anesthesia used in childbirth, given through the spinal canal
cephalhematoma	subcutaneous swelling found on the head of an infant several days after delivery
cephalic	referring to the head
cervical dilation	the cervical os and the cervical canal widen from less than 1 centimeter to approximately 10 centimeters
chloasma	brownish pigmentation over the bridge of the nose
chorion	one of the two uterine membranes closest to the intrauterine wall
Leopold's maneuvers	series of four maneuvers designed to allow the examiner to determine fetal presentation and position
mastitis	inflammation of the breast
neonatal mortality rate	number of deaths of infants in the first 28 days of life per 1,000 live births
neonate	infant from birth through the first 28 days of life
neonatology	the specialty that focuses on the management of high-risk conditions of the newborn
omphalitis	infection of the umbilicus
omphalocele	congential herniation of abdominal contents into the base of the umbilicus
outlet dystocia	inadequate pelvic size, causing the fetal head to be pushed backward toward the coccyx, making delivery of head difficult
ovum	female reproductive cell; egg
oxygen toxicity	serious, sometimes irreversible damage to pulmonary capillary endothelium associated with excessive levels of oxygen therapy
oxytocics	drugs that stimulate uterine contractions
oxytocin	hormone normally produced by the posterior pituitary, responsible for stimulation of uterine contractions and the release of milk into the lactiferous ducts
oxytocin challenge test (OCT)	also called the contraction stress test (CCST), the test evaluates the circulatory and respiratory status of the fetoplacental unit
palpation	use of fingers or hands to manually perform assessment
perforation of the uterus	a hole made in the uterus
perineum	the area of tissue between the anus and vagina in the female
periodic breathing	sporadic episodes of apnea, not associated with cyanosis, lasting about 10 seconds
persistent pulmonary hypertension	a neonatal syndrome secondary to pulmonary hypertension; seen in preterm but more frequently in full-term and postmature infants
phenylketonuria (PKU)	a recessive hereditary metabolic error that causes the buildup of phenylalanine, leading to mental retardation,

	brain damage, light pigmentation and other growth deformities. It is treated with a low-phenylalanine diet
phlebitis	inflammation of a vein
phototherapy	treatment of newborn jaundice by exposure to natural or special artificial light
physiologic jaundice	harmless condition caused by the normal reduction of red blood cells, occurs usually between the second and fifth day after birth, peaking on the fifth to seventh day, and disappearing between the seventh and tenth day.
placenta previa	improper implantation of the placenta on the lower uterine segment. Classification of type is based on closeness to the cervical os: total—completely covers the os; partial—covers a portion of the os; marginal—in close proximity to the os
preterm infant	any infant born before 37 weeks' gestation
preterm labor	labor beginning before the 37th week of gestation
primipara	a woman who has given birth to her first child
postmature infant	a newborn that is overly developed or that is more than 42 weeks' gestation
postnatal	occurring after birth
precipitous delivery	unduly rapid progression of labor
preeclampsia	toxemia of pregnancy; characterized by hypertension, albuminuria, and edema
pregnancy-induced hypertension (PIH)	a hypertensive disorder including preeclampsia and identified by the three cardinal signs: hypertension, edema, and proteinuria
prolapsed cord	umbilical cord that becomes compressed in the vagina before the fetus is delivered, resulting in emergency situation for the fetus
prolonged labor	labor lasting more than 24 hours
puerperium	the period after completion of the third stage of labor until involution of the uterus is complete at about 6 weeks
quickening	the first fetal movements felt by the pregnant woman, usually between 16 and 18 weeks' gestation
rales	an abnormal respiratory sound caused by air passing through fluid in the alveoli and bronchioles
regional anesthesia	injection of local anesthetic
rhonchi	coarse, abnormal auscultatory sounds
saddle block anesthesia	sensory and motor anesthesia of the buttocks, perineum, and inner aspects of the thighs, produced by spinal or intrathecal injection
show	a pinkish mucous discharge from the vagina that may occur a few hours to a few days before the onset of labor
spina bifida occulta	a defect in the vertebrae of the spinal column without protrusion of neural components
subinvolution	failure of a part to return to its normal size
surfactant	a surface-active mixture of secreted lipoproteins caused by *Candida albicans*, in the alveoli and air passages; it reduces surface tension of pulmonary fluids and contributes to the elasticity of lung tissue
tachycardia	abnormally rapid heart rate
tachypnea	excessively rapid respirations

term infant a liveborn infant at 38 to 42 weeks' gestation

thromboembolus thrombotic material or clot within the vein

tocodynamometer external device that can be used to estimate uterine contraction pressures during labor

umbilical cord the structure connecting the placenta to the umbilicus of the fetus through which the fetus receives nutrition and eliminates wastes

urinary meatus external opening of the urethra

uterus the hollow muscular organ in which the fertilized egg is implanted and in which the developing fetus is nourished until birth

vagina the musculomembranous tube located between the external genitals and the uterus

varicose veins permanently distended veins

vasectomy surgical removal of a portion of the vas deferens

Index

Note: Page numbers followed by *t* indicate tables.